Nurse Educators and Politics

Nurse Educators and Politics

Sondra Z. Koff

State University of New York Press

Published by
State University of New York Press, Albany

For information, address State University of New York Press,
90 State Street, Suite 700, Albany, NY 12207

Production by Kelli Williams
Marketing by Susan Petrie

Library of Congress Cataloging-in-Publication Data

Koff, Sondra Z.
    Nurse educators and politics / Sondra Z. Koff.
       p. cm.
    Includes bibliographical references and index.
    ISBN 0-7914-6073-8 (alk. paper)
       1. Nursing. 2. Nursing—Political aspects. 3. Nursing—Study and
teaching. I. Title.

RT4.K645   2004
610.73'071'173—dc22

                                                          2004045255

10 9 8 7 6 5 4 3 2 1

For
Ida and Charles
Prime Movers and Shakers

Contents

Preface

Over time conversations with friends who are nurses and my experiences on health care boards that included nurses revealed a striking lack of political consciousness on the part of representatives of the nursing profession. This shortcoming and its high cost to the profession were startling to me, even though I was aware that professional leaders for some time have been writing about the price of political insensitivity and the minimal response to their warnings. My curiosity was stimulated and this book is the result.

In an attempt to understand the category's behavior, this effort focuses on a primary socialization agent to the profession: nursing faculty members. Their culture, values and role modeling are critical determinants of the behavior of nurses on the political stage. Given the sparse interaction between the social sciences and nursing, my intention was to write a work of use to two constituencies: students of the social sciences and health care. I wanted to familiarize those in health care with certain basic political science concepts and to expose those in the social sciences to some fundamentals of the nursing profession. I hope I have achieved my goal.

In writing this book I was fortunate to be able to draw on the talents of several capable individuals. Two persons who might have been coauthors had not distance, new responsibilities, and a change in career paths occurred must be singled out for attention. I had the pleasure of sharing many a dinner and hours of telephone conversation with Mary Germain, associate professor, State University of New

York, Downstate Medical Center, College of Nursing. We discussed at length many of the topics covered in this book. She was important to the undertaking in its initial stages and especially in the development and distribution of the questionnaire that served as the basis for this study. James Wehrli, a fellow political scientist and close friend, played a significant role in the early research facet of the project. He was imaginative, exacting and thorough. I am also grateful to him for his assistance in the preparation of the data for analysis.

Others have been of aid in diverse ways. Cathryne A. Welch, former executive director of the New York State Nurses Association and now the executive director of the Foundation of the New York State Nurses Association, has been a special friend for many years as well as a mentor. She has served as a sounding board for many of the ideas in this book and interpreted for me some of the survey results. Also Marie Reed, former executive director of the American Nurses Credentialing Center, lent me her ear and shared her valuable insights on the national nursing scene. My husband, Stephen Koff, also a political scientist, had a significant role in the preparation of this work. In addition to his active encouragement, he did so many things that made this project much easier and more fun than it might have been. Even though he works in a different field, he provided valuable observations and ideas. Playing devil's advocate, he proficiently used his penchant to ask the right questions. His perspective was extremely useful. Ida Benderson, volunteer extraordinaire, is responsible for launching my contacts with the world of nursing. To her I am indebted because these have provided me not only many hours of hard work, but much enjoyment and many rewards. I must also recognize those nurse educators who took the time to complete the survey instrument and those who contacted me with their personal comments. The United University Professions provided a research grant. Professional colleagues, on a variety of health care boards on which I have served as a public member, have been more than willing to entertain my ideas, respond to my questions, and share their experiences. Never have I been treated as an outsider or intruder.

Being able to pursue a study of the Italian nursing profession as I was writing this book has afforded me the opportunity to develop professional relationships with practitioners in that nation who quickly became friends. Conversations with Tina Ernesta Galli, Lida Intrieri, JoAnn Lindsay, Anna Maria Olivieri, and Angela Panini have provided a wealth of discussion. Their questions about the American nursing profession forced me to think about it in another context. Responses to these questions and to mine about Italian nursing indicate that many of the points raised in this work are applicable to the Italian scene. I am also indebted to the late Piero Moggi, a professor, physician, and maverick who was fervently concerned about the consequences of nurses' political insensitivity.

In spite of the abundance of aid I received, I assume full responsibility for the contents of this work and hope to have made a contribution to the improvement of our knowledge of the nursing profession.

Sondra Z. Koff

Chapter 1

Nursing and the Political Arena

What is the future of nursing as a profession? What will its role be in the health care delivery system and on the social and political stages? These questions for many a year have provided a basis for discussion. In this debate, overwhelming calls of pessimism issued by members of the profession have been heard loud and clear. In the words of one practitioner:

> Is this the beginning of the end of nursing? Impossible some will say. Impossible because of the numbers of nurses and the invaluable service they render to society. Think again. Peter Drucker points out that at the turn of the century the largest populations of workers were farmers and live-in servants. Ninety years later, these groups barely exist. Although farmers and domestic servants were everywhere, as a class, they were invisible. Drucker attributes their invisibility to the fact they were not organized as a group. As a class, nurses may be more visible inasmuch as they are organized. However, they remain vulnerable. Their work remains invisible to far too many. The invisibility of nurses may lead to our profession's demise. (Gottlieb, 1996, p. 4)

These strong words present a desperate situation. Yet we all know that this knowledge-based group, being essential to the operation of the health care delivery system, will survive. The important question is: In what form will it survive? The response, in part, will be decided, like other professional issues, by the interplay of political forces and the resulting public policies. Nurse leaders are in general agreement that nursing's continuous evolution as a truly autonomous profession is inextricably bound to its ability to influence policy development and to evidence a positive public image of nursing as an essential societal service.

The concept of power and its distribution and use are concerns of many groups, including professions. It is generally acknowledged that the most important part of the professionalization process, ". . . an attempt to translate one order of scarce resources—special knowledge and skills—into another—social and economic rewards" (Larson, 1977, p. xvii), is gaining and maintaining power and control. Power is defined as the ability to influence or persuade decision makers to act in a way congruent with desired outcomes. Professional power has dual aspects. It may be sought and exerted at a local or parochial level, that is, internally, or in a national or cosmopolitan setting, that is, externally. The nursing profession has not always enjoyed access to the external, broader, societal dimension of power and, consequently, it was forced to focus most of its efforts in a narrower fashion, internally on the profession. Internal power had to compensate for external power.

In comparison to other professionals, especially physicians, little has been written on the topic of power, politics and policy related to nursing. Although the profession has engaged in the power game at the cosmopolitan level, it has been demonstrated again and again that nurses have not been adept at politics. Their political efforts, with rare exception, have been casual, nebulous, and lacking in continuity. There has been a failure to recognize their potential impact on the political arena and the significance of the nursing profession as an interest group. Cathryne A. Welch (1985), a prominent commentator on the profession, has appropriately written:

> As a profession, nursing has not been a major determinant
> of health policy in this country.

> Predominantly, nursing has been in a reactionary or re-
> sponsive state versus the creative role with respect to de-
> signing health policy. Frankly . . . nursing has stood on the
> periphery of both power and politics for so long as a result
> of its inability to use its own force in the formulation of
> health policy. (p. 107)

This judgment is not atypical.

Being the largest of the health care professions and consisting, according to the Bureau of Health Professions, of 2.6 million registered
nurses and, thus, representing a significant majority of American
health care providers, and accounting for the largest noncapital portion of health care institutional budgets, nursing should have been
more influential than it has been in the making of health care policy.
In spite of their numbers, nurses have experienced difficulty in chan-
neling their strength to achieve status, recognition and power. Historically, they have had limited power in the health care delivery system
as well as in the political arena. They have been isolated from political, social and economic power. Never having been able to capitalize
on its knowledge, skills, numerical advantage and key role in the
health care delivery system for utilization of power on the political
stage, the profession has often been referred to as a "sleeping giant."

One element important to the development of political competence is faculty role modeling of the knowledge, attitudes, and behaviors associated with successfully impacting the political system.
Perhaps nursing education has not demonstrated the significance of
participation in policy development and nursing faculty have not
served as critical role models. It may be that the profession has fallen
far short of its potential impact on health care policy, in part, because
of the manner in which socialization agents have functioned.

Inherent in the preparation of the professional practitioner of
nursing is this concept of socialization, meaning the learning of values, attitudes, morals, knowledge and skills. One of the skills that
nursing education programs, especially baccalaureate and higher-degree ones, profess to transmit to their students is the ability to influence health care policy development in general and, in particular, that
related to nursing. Faculty role modeling is a significant factor in the
creation of this competency. Data from the nursing literature suggests, however, that although nursing graduates, especially those with

a baccalaureate degree, value professional autonomy and leadership, many may not see change and its implementation through active participation in professional associations and policy making as part of their professional role. If such is the case, labeling these graduates "change agents" may be a misnomer with significant adverse repercussions for the profession of nursing.

The graduates' ambivalence toward the importance of professional organizational affiliations and participation in policy development may reflect the knowledge, attitudes, and behaviors role modeled by the nursing faculty to which they are exposed. In view of this, it is imperative to examine the role modeling that nurse faculty members exhibit relative to the profession's role in policy development. To date this has not been done. This work discusses the role of nurses in the political process. More specifically, it examines nurse educators' attitudes toward political participation and the behavior these professionals exhibit relative to political and organizational activism. The study is based on an extensive questionnaire administered to full-time faculty members in baccalaureate and higher-degree programs in the state of New York. Research objectives were threefold: (1) to examine the nurse educators' participation in professional, political, and other organizations; (2) to examine their knowledge of and attitudes toward select professional concerns; and (3) to examine their actual involvement in the promotion of policies and candidates supportive to nursing. All of these relate to how nursing faculty members serve as role models for their students.

Professions, however, cannot be understood in terms of the current balance of social relations. One cannot study any given profession without studying its context. Present-day behavior has its roots in various stages and facets of professional history (Tousijn, 1997) containing many forces referred to as determinants. These critical elements forming over time in a profession's development influence the conduct of its practitioners today. Many factors have been used to explain nurses' limited power. In addition to history and its broad social formations, these include the state and its organization, gender composition of the profession, religious and military influences, professional closure, education, the work setting, remuneration, and culture and socialization to the profession. Before pursuing the main focus of this work, I will briefly discuss each of these elements so that the reader will be able to relate the major theme to a broader perspective.

Politics is not new to nursing. Gains for the
been minimized, in part because throughout its his
exercised power as individuals and not collectively.
visionary and capable nursing leaders who, exerti
nally, were consummate politicians. However, they
number. Most leaders, having a restricted vision of power, have been
internalists. Nursing in the course of its development as a profession
has constantly been in a position of being controlled by a variety of
outside forces. Thus, it has experienced a long history of dependency
in major health care decisions. Politically, the profession has been recognized primarily at times of crisis. It has been essentially dismissed
as a significant political actor.

Nurses themselves, leaders and otherwise, have admitted and
complained that their counsel has rarely been sought in health care
planning. In part, this situation resulted because, although organized
nursing considers itself professional, the public has held this profession in a different regard from that of medicine or law. Thus, it has
not been consulted on issues of public policy in the same manner as
the other professions. In general, when there are questions concerning health care matters, the advice of physicians and hospital administrators has been sought. And if solicited, the counsel of nurses has
usually not been taken as seriously as that of more influential constituencies. A recent development in the profession is increased interest in the public policy arena and greater recognition by other
players. Influence, to date, however, has lagged behind enhanced interest and recognition.

THE STATE AND ITS ORGANIZATION

Different types of knowledge-based groups result from diverse
social and political environments, a major component of which is
the nature of the nation-state and its organization. Use of the word
state should not be confused with the subnational unit of government in the United States, that is, New York State, Maine,
Wyoming, and so on. As used here, "nation-state" refers to a sover-
eign unit whose constitution distributes power to the various institutions and whose policies are determined by its agent, government.

role of the nation-state has been paramount in the evolution of various professions.

> [It] has granted legitimacy to the professions by, for example, licensing professional activity, and setting standards of practice to ensure public safety and protection. The state has also acted as a guarantor of professional education, not least by giving public funds for academic education and research . . . the state has extended its support for the professions by paying for the services rendered to the public by professional experts. (Hellberg, Saks, & Benoit, 1999, p. 2)

A monopoly over the provision of a particular service, the ideal of any knowledge-based group, can only be granted by the state. The role of the state and sectors within it fluctuate according to the values that dominate at a given point in history. Professional activities continually change in content and legitimation. Legitimacy is of particular importance to professions. It justifies what they do and how they do it. It denotes approval and establishes that their activities reflect cultural values and norms. Professions, having a distinctive relationship with the state, explain their professional position at any point in time as a result of their encounters with it (Abbott, 1988; Macdonald, 1995). In their pursuit of monopoly and privilege, professions cannot avoid the state. They must use it to support the basis of their professional claim.

A basic distinction between nation-states is that of the welfare state, as exemplified by countries in continental Europe, and the liberal state as in the case of the United States. In the former, the concept of governance features the promotion and maintenance of social goals such as income support, including pensions and child subsidies; housing; and health care and social services provision. Citizens are endowed with a broad array of legally guaranteed social and economic rights. Economic, physical, mental and cultural security is facilitated for the citizenry by services forthcoming from the public sector and paid for by taxation. In the liberal state as it exists today, the claims of rights of individuals are not as broad as in the welfare state and, thus, the social agenda is much more restricted. Many of the same goods and services that are forthcoming from the public sector in the welfare state are purchased in the liberal state on the market from diverse professional practitioners by citizens as customers or clients.

Not only does this distinction between states bear consequences for the role and position of the citizen, but it also impacts on the role and development of knowledge-based groups. The professions regulate the market and are regulated by the market in the liberal state, whereas in the welfare state, professions regulate the law and are regulated by it. The allocation of social goods in the liberal state is realized by means of the supply and demand of the market, and in the welfare state by means of law. Professions have important but diverse roles in the distribution of social goods depending on the nature of the state. Moreover, they have a different kind of relationship with the state depending, again, on its type.

The driving force for the development of professions in continental Europe and especially Scandinavia was principally the demands and needs of the welfare state. Professional development was linked to the development of citizen rights. As the state expanded its public sector activities and, thus, services to the citizenry, the development of the individual professions reflected the ambitions that the state had for them. For example, in the Scandinavian nations, the state promoted expansion of the health care system. As it has grown within the confines of the welfare state, so has nursing. In this case the state has served as a significant source of legitimation. Having a critical role in its activities, nursing achieved social legitimacy. There is a relationship between professional power and citizens' rights. Furthermore, these professions have become identified with the state in such a way that they perform a moderating function between the state and its citizenry. They occupy a critical and sensitive spot. Being in service of the state and firmly implanted in the public sector, health care professions, and specifically nursing, have been assigned various responsibilities that the welfare state has toward its citizens. In exchange for carrying out these duties, the state initiated authorization for the professions to perform certain tasks and offered aid in establishing professional closure or territoriality, a demarcation of professional boundaries and responsibilities (Bertilsson, 1990; Brante, 1999; Elzinga, 1990; Hellberg, 1990). In essence, in the welfare or interventionist state, professionalization evolves "from above," that is, within the state. The state and the professions are joined in a partnership in which both pursue their own interests.

The situation varies considerably in the liberal state with its laissez-faire philosophical foundation based on the notion that the government that governs best is the one that governs least. The restricted role of the state has meant that the principal determinant of the development of the nursing profession in the United States has been private-sector enterprise and not the state, as in continental Europe. Professions, not being in service of the state, established themselves apart from it. The formation of monopolistic practitioner organizations operating on the market for services was important. These structures, lending status to individual groups, assumed the initiative and approached the state to support their power of monopolization and self-regulation over their members. Thus, the liberal state, as opposed to its welfare counterpart, is a passive recipient of stimuli from aspiring knowledge-based groups. It does not initiate, but rather reacts. Moreover, the politics of professional development and projection also differ in the two state models. In the welfare state, conflict centers on bureaucratic position and in its liberal counterpart, the struggles are for decentralized market regulation associations. Both models have affected professional identities and work conditions (Castro, 1999; Collins, 1990; Fielding & Portwood, 1980; Larson, 1990; Torstendahl, 1990). In essence, the shape of the state has had significant connotations for many facets of nursing's collective development.

GENERAL

GENDER

Throughout their history, the values of a patriarchal society have been built into the institutions and practices of the caring professions, such as nursing. Being embedded in a gendered world, in the sense that nursing is composed largely of women, that profession has been impacted negatively in its attempt to leave its mark on the public agenda and health care institutions. There is a link between gender, status and power. Structured features of the profession, regarded primarily as a female one and as an extension of domestic service, can be related to its gender composition. Caregivers, like women in general, have been defined and delimited by patriarchal custom and male authority. This, in part, accounts for the low esteem assigned to nursing. The lack of leadership in the profession has been explained by reference to nurses' social orientation as women. In fact, the role of nursing in the health field is the epitome of the female role in American society. The status of nursing at any point in time reflects the status of women. Both are manifestations of prevailing sex-role norms. For example, after valiant service in World War I, nursing's professional image declined dramatically. Most nurses were unmarried and thus lacked the prestige that marriage brought in the society of that era. Nursing problems are a part of the larger question of women's social, economic, sexual and political bondage. There are many connections between the subordinated status of women and of women in the nursing profession (Ashley, 1977; Capuzzi, 1980; James, 1985; Lewis, 1985; Roberts & Group, 1995).

Davies (1995) posits that gender divisions are basic to all social structures and gender codes of masculinity and femininity pervade organizations in such a way that they and their interrelationships are gendered. She argues: "Starting from assumptions, such as these, what appears initially as disconnected personal discontents of women as nurses gradually transmutes into the collective dilemmas of nurses as women—the dilemmas, in other words, of gender" (p. ix). In short, gender fashions the way people relate to each other and it pervades their institutions, including those of work and politics.

Not accorded full professional status, the nurse is perceived as a female who has a "job" rather than a profession or a career. This, in turn trivializing the practitioner's work and belittling those who perform it, creates doubts about the profession's leadership and its members (Davies, 1995). Hierarchical relationships within the health care system reflect this situation. Consequently, it has been extremely difficult for nurses to gain influence external to their profession. It is generally assumed that "women are a subgroup, that 'man's world' is the real world, that patriarchy is equivalent to culture and culture to patriarchy . . ." (Code, 1988, p. 20). In the patriarchal health care system, thought structures and social policies have dictated a particular and subordinate status for women in the "man's world." Given the traditional gendered nature of the health care professions, the predominantly female profession of nursing has been less privileged than those dominated by males.

The sheer number of women in the profession has placed a brake on the extent to which it could make a bid for power in the political and professional arenas. Despite being a heavily female world, nursing is not a united world founded on gender. This fragmentation complicates the situation even more. One of the profession's many divisions is based on age. As in most professions, there is a gulf between the older and younger generations, which in the case of nursing, was congruent with a schism between nurse leaders and regular nurses. Moreover, marital status has divided the practitioners. For example, as far as leadership is concerned, until after World War II there were almost no married women influential in the internal affairs of nursing. However, some leaders had been married and widowed or divorced. Also, at one time, married women were not accepted into most nursing schools because of the conflict between having to live in the hospital and maintaining an outside home. In additon, many work sites preferred singles and some were legally restricted to unmarried women. Working conditions definitely favored single females. Eventually, barriers based on marital status disappeared and it was possible to combine marriage, family, and a career without being ostracized. Divisions such as these, in addition to severe professional ones that will be presented throughout this work, have plagued the profession, especially in its bid for power (Goodman-Draper, 1995). Nurses are perceived as having many positive qualities, but the list does not include power. It remains to be seen whether the profession's attempt to achieve increased power will materialize or not. Unfortunately, ". . . perceptions and images of nurses are processed . . . according to ingrained, gender-based, stereotyped schemata, totally opposite to images of power and influence" (Roberts & Group, 1995, p. 292).

Being essentially a female profession, and the largest group of professional women in the United States, it could be expected that nursing would have connected immediately and intimately with feminist concerns, especially the struggle for the franchise and the women's movement. However, the profession as well as its individual members were slow to embrace these elements. The two constituencies, the female and nursing worlds, had diverse foci. Nursing in the latter 1800s was primarily preoccupied with professional growth and control. It applied social feminist activism to its own professional agenda (Lewenson, 1993). It was concerned with issues specific to the profession, such as autonomy, self-control, work schedules, pay equity and professional equality. On the other hand, the women's movement had broader horizons and more general concerns relating to work opportunities, education and political rights for women. Moreover, when, in 1907, the suffrage movement re-emerged with the founding of the Equality League of Self-Supporting Women, few nurses were quick to grasp its message. In addition, there were strained relations between the profession and the National Woman's Party that was active on the political stage from 1913 to 1920 and an important force in obtaining women's right to vote.

Nursing leadership, from a practical perspective, eventually became aware of the importance of the franchise to realization of professional objectives. As these leaders struggled for state licensure, their inability to vote for such a change underscored the significance of female suffrage. Perceived as a guarantor of women's rights in the home and at work, the vote symbolized personal and professional freedom. A new stance was consequently assumed by the profession at the 1915 gathering of the governing body of the American Nurses Association (ANA), the principal representative body of the profession. Previous opposition to women's suffrage was overturned. This new orientation was congruent with the spirit of the late nineteenth and early twentieth-century women's movement. It was realized that nursing and feminists had overlapping and complementary interests. Nursing organizations allied with other women's groups in their attempt to improve the social, political, and economic conditions of females. The nursing profession moved from its parochial professional concerns toward a more extensive and active role in the social reforms of the Progressive era.

If members of the profession were hesitant to endorse the franchise, they were equally hesitant to support the Equal Rights Amendment (ERA) that was placed on the public agenda in 1923, immediately after women were given the right to vote. Nursing was as divided as feminists on this issue that was supported only by a small minority. Opposition centered on the fear that implementation would result in the invalidation of all social legislation protecting women achieved as the result of fierce battles during the Progressive years. Fifty years after its introduction, the ERA was approved by Congress, but it was not ratified for lack of votes. Although nursing was heavily involved in these two controversial struggles, it was not in the vanguard of either, nor did it assert itself in a leadership capacity (Palmer, 1983).

The alliance between nursing and the women's movement has always had its uneasy moments. However, it was most fragile when feminist activities in the broader society intensified in the early 1960s (Feldman & Lewenson, 2000). Failing to acknowledge the ties between the two constituencies at the start of the last century, women's groups put down nursing. These feminists were externalists. They knew little and cared little about the internal world of the profession. Basically they disregarded it. Even though they were promoting the advancement of women in male-defined professions that systematically oppress females, they did not consider as worthy of attention the political, professional and personal potential women created in nursing. In part, the discrepancy between feminists and nursing resulted from a lack of, and incorrect, knowledge of the profession that generated many misunderstandings.

Nurses were severely chastised for their promulgation of negative female stereotypes. Feminists regarded them as the epitome of woman's servile role. Moreover, they pointed to a large body of professional literature, penned by nurses, that affirmed the male definition and domination of the profession along with the systemic oppression of its members. Nurses were thought to be the victims of a totally male-defined system, considered to be the opium of the feminists, and in essence, the professional response was labeled weak. Nursing, it was charged, had succumbed to oppressed-group behavior and was imitating what it viewed as powerful, that which is male. Not only were nurses accused of identifying with the oppressor, symbolized by physicians and administrators, but it was charged with a form of antifeminist self-aggression. This disregard for nurses is evident in the feminist and working women's literature. There is very little material focusing on the profession. The largest single group of female workers in the nation is barely mentioned in connection with politics and the women's movement (Archer & Goehner, 1982; Lewenson, 1993; Lynaugh & Brush, 1996). These accusations took their toll on nursing. Many potential students selected other occupational directions and as a reaction to the lack of respect and questioning of their worth by other professionals and society at large, many nurses deserted the profession. Within it morale dramatically declined and practitioners were generally overcome with a sense of powerlessness and lack of self-esteem, significant obstacles to assertiveness external to the profession.

In spite of the tense relationship and lack of collaboration between feminists and nurses, some practitioners believed that the women's movement could be used as an instrument for the advancement of the profession. Thus, some prime feminist nursing leaders effectively linked the liberation of women with that of nursing. This was done most capably by Wilma Scott Heide, who served as the head of the National Organization for Women. Nurse scholars have positively evaluated the impact of feminism on their profession, especially as it relates to professional development and the utilization of power and politics. In addition, the women's movement is credited with putting nursing economic issues, such as remuneration, chauvinistic treatment, and less-than-desirable working conditions, as well as the importance of self-fulfillment, on center stage. It is generally acknowledged that feminism could and did contribute more to nursing than nursing offered feminism (Lerner, 1985; Roberts & Group, 1995).

RELIGION AND THE MILITARY

Professional attitudes result from specific historical situations. In the case of nursing, the environment in which the profession developed, colored at times by religion and the military, provides, in part, an explanation for its failure to realize its potential strength in the political arena. Religion has been important to the history of nursing. The profession, embedded in Judeo-Christian institutions, is a product of a long religious tradition. Given the Bible's emphasis on care and healing, it was natural for nursing to become a major responsibility of the church in the early Christian era as evidenced by the monastic care and concern for the ill. Providing training and care, many religious orders, both Catholic and Protestant, were closely associated with nursing, first abroad and then eventually in the United States. This religious orientation resulted in a confusing overlap of religious vocation or calling and intellectual and personal commitment for nurses identified with these religious institutions. The seeds of asceticism, self-abnegation, obedience to authority, and strict discipline were sowed as ideals essential to nursing practice. They became the watchwords of the profession and have continued to exert influence until this day, although in altered form. Not only has religion impacted the personal concerns of nurses, but, in part, religious movements account for the feminization of the profession. Religious imagery has also had a part in the domination of women. There are images of female submissiveness in the New and Old Testaments and these have been employed to justify the general dominance of males over females. Thus, as far as the nursing profession is concerned, this religious sex-role imagery legitimated the professional order of female subordination to the male (Brown, Nolan, & Crawford, 2000; LaChat, 1988). These religious tendencies are not conducive to participatory and assertive behavior.

Wars have also been an important factor in the development of the nursing profession. Military nursing orders had their origins in the Crusades, the military expeditions undertaken by Christians in the eleventh through the thirteenth centuries to take the Holy Land from the Moslems. This was part of the penetration of the military into the profession. Military influence yielded results similar to the religious. The military spirit even pervaded early nursing education that, reflecting Florence Nightingale's model for the army medical service in the Crimea, emphasized dedication to duty and obedience to superiors, both qualities expected of an exemplary soldier. Military influence continued to develop in innumerable wars throughout the world and professional nursing eventually became a feature of the military establishment.

PROFESSIONAL CLOSURE

Whether nursing is a profession or not has served as a source of lively and bitter debate. Some authorities consider it a profession, although a relatively young one. On the other hand, there are those who affirm that professional status remains to be obtained. In this study, 76% of the participants believed that nursing was a profession as opposed to a quasi-profession or an occupation. Although the literature concerned with professions is vast and contains much disagreement over the variables that are considered crucial in distinguishing occupations from professions, there appears to be consensus on the characteristic of autonomy. This element is perceived as being critical to professional status. The core of any profession is control of tasks, which is determined by the culture and established by competitive claims in the political arena. The potential for autonomy varies as occupations change over time in terms of skill content and cultural significance. Thus, the concept of territoriality is important to professions.

As noted previously, gaining and maintaining power and control is an important facet of the professionalization project. Much of the sociological literature on professions stresses this struggle for power and privilege. A part of this effort is territoriality or closure, ". . . a process through which an occupation controls entry into itself . . ." (Walby & Greenwell, 1994, p. 63). It ". . . involves a set of practices whereby an occupation creates a monopoly over its skills by both controlling entry to training and membership, and by preventing others from practicing that trade who have not acquired recognized membership" (Walby & Greenwell, p. 63). A profession must establish boundaries to its knowledge and occupational area and methods of protecting its territory from attack by those persons external to it. Clearly some professions have been more successful in this endeavor than others. Nursing has been less adept than other knowledge-based groups. Various strategies and instruments are used to achieve closure, the major purpose of which is to maximize rewards by limiting access to resources and opportunities to a restricted set of eligible persons. (Ramprogus, 1995). Education, legislation and professional associations are the most common tools employed.

Education produces professional skills and the knowledge base of the profession. It puts in place a particular preparation based on a systematic body of theory allowing for the acquisition of a professional culture. Its content coincides with professional expansion, attacks, potential and real, to the material base of the profession, and demands for access to professional services from previously disenfranchised groups. Moreover, its curricula encompass and legitimate partial versions of professional work and interests (Atkinson, 1985; Dubar, 1991). Licensure, practice acts, and other legislation secure professional jurisdictional limitations. Reflecting the federalist distribution of power in the United States, these legislative measures vary from one individual state to another. For example, each features Nurse Practice Acts that result from the police power granted to it by the national government to protect the safety of its population. Although they differ from state to state in terms of specifics, most define the nursing function and describe educational requirements for entry into practice, the licensure process and exemptions from it, scope of practice, composition and selection of the state board of nursing, disciplinary procedure and reciprocity. Usually the practice is discussed in such a way that it allows for the necessary freedom of interpretation of the law to account for new and innovative techniques and future conditions of practice.

Professions are part of a social system with constant interaction and competition affecting all, some for better and some for worse. Changes in the circumstances of one profession usually impact on the position of one or more of the others. All are interdependent and the basis of their identity is subject to modification. The shape of knowledge-based groups is ever changing because territoriality is a dynamic concept. It can be expanded, restricted, or withdrawn when the professional environment demands change. Consequently, professional associations are important because they allow an occupational group to promote its interests and to shield itself from competition.

All of these closure tools, being organized on a legal basis and consisting of a mosaic of constitutional clauses, legislative enactments, judicial interpretations, and agency rules, are intimately identified with politics. Closure is definitely subject to political struggle. Moreover, the existence of distinct models of closure demonstrates professionalization is a historically specific concept. In addition to politics, closure is closely affected by the profession's past, its specific activity and the workplace (Burau, 1999; Larson, 1990; Saks 1999). Territoriality is important to a profession and motivation to achieve it is great. Status, material rewards, the legitimation of authority, prestige, power, ambition to create elitism and monopoly of service, a claim to autonomy, upward social mobility, and desire to assume more exclusive functions all provide the stimulus to pursue it.

As noted, closure has been difficult for the nursing profession. Most evident is the fact that its efforts resulted in a subordinate position for nurses vis-à-vis physicians, ". . . the encirclement of women within a related but distinct sphere of competence in an occupational division of labor and . . . their . . . subordination to male-dominated occupations" (Witz, 1992, pp. 47–48). The early state medical practice acts were penned in the nineteenth century before any of the other health occupations had practice acts. These acts made physicians responsible for all health care. Thus, in the next century, when other practice acts were drawn up, physicians' territory was challenged. For dentistry and veterinary medicine, this was not a problem. Their independence did not encroach on physicians. However, in the case of nursing and some other professions, it was difficult to create a niche (B. Bullough, 1983, 1994). In fact, the profession is still negotiating psychological separation from medicine and its boundaries vis-à-vis the more expansive medical practice acts. This negotiation is more arduous than it might have been because nurses acquiesced to the boundaries originally created by physicians and to the expansive definition of their prerogatives. Nursing's present-day attempt to expand its clinical authority has received diverse responses depending on the particular state involved. The reduction of the historically strict physician supervision and use of protocols has been especially difficult. Challenges from the state medical societies have been formidable. Several factors work against a general victory for nursing whose battle, some argue, was lost when the production of physicians dramatically increased and the profession was not aggressive in carving out a larger space in the health care system. With a surplus of doctors, the prospect for enlarged scope of nursing practice is not favorable. Moreover, another difficulty is finding allies when government and business have a single interest: cost containment.

Although nursing's boundaries have always clashed with those of medicine, the recent decline in the latter's power in the health care system and in the political arena may not be enough to fully enhance nursing's professional status. It might be that a change in gender ideology is needed for promotion of greater nurse autonomy. A recent survey of British and American medical students (Levinson, McCranie, Scambler, & Scambler, 1995) did not indicate more general support for role sharing between physicians and nurses. However, female respondents were more sympathetic to the notion. In any case, such jurisdictional disputes are major determinants of professional history. In fact, they provide the impetus and pattern to organizational developments (Abbott, 1988; E. Greenwood, 1972; Manley, 1995).

Given the dynamic nature of closure, knowledge-based groups must continually maneuver for position in the professional arena to maintain or enhance their power and to meet the competition for professional space. Nursing's task in this regard is more severe than that of many of its professional counterparts, due to its failure to clearly and forcefully stake out its turf from early in its development and define its special role in the delivery of health care. Not having convinced society and the professional health care realm that nobody else can carry out its work without endangering the patient, the importance and nonsubstitutability of nursing activity have not been demonstrated. Nurses have been challenged by new occupations claiming professional mandate and by the increasingly sophisticated demands of the consumers.

There is competition from others who display an overlap of boundaries of practice. Other practitioners, whose skills and training overlap, are ready to provide similar, substitute or complementary services, whether they are dieticians, laboratory or operating room technicians, social workers, physician assistants, psychologists, occupational or physical therapists, orderlies, licensed practical nurses, financial management officers, or clerks. These folks can offer their substitute services on a legal basis. It is noteworthy that physicians have no such legal substitutes. An examination of the state nurse practice acts demonstrates that professional nurses have overlapping functions with these other health care providers. Moreover, the professional nurse is often brought into direct conflict with the physician because of direct medical supervision requirements and those mandating medical permission (Levi, 1980, 1995). The profession has not been able to use autonomy to prevent outside interference and supervision.

A major problem confronting nursing today is that of functional redundancy. There is no task that nurses perform that is not also carried out by another type of practitioner. To eliminate functional redundancy, the nursing profession will have to define its domain in such a way that its boundaries are distinct from those of other health care groups, achieve internal consensus on its unique role and rally the forces of its political power network to implement closure. A knowledge base distinct from social knowledge in general and the establishment of a special claim to it are essential ingredients of professional status and power.

Nursing occupies a sensitive and uncomfortable position in the health care delivery system from which it is difficult to respond to challenges to its territoriality. Given the role of medicine in the hierarchy, nursing faces a fierce obstacle if it attempts to move upward and invade the medical arena. It is equally unwelcome if its upward movement is toward administration, another male-dominated world. Lateral actions are no more comfortable in that the territory on both sides is occupied by professions with overlapping boundaries to whom nursing over time has been relinquishing tasks. There is also pressure from below from support workers. The profession in this structure is a lonely crusader and has few friends. This is the special dilemma that nursing faces in terms of closure. It is especially severe because the profession lacks control over its labor supply in general and particularly over cycles of shortage and surplus (Levi, 1995; Walby & Greenwell, 1994). The professional complex as it relates to closure continues to be permeated with conflict. Its battles take place at the workplace, in public opinion, and on the political stage.

EDUCATION

Education has played an important part in readying women for particular work roles at the same time that it differentiated the female labor force along class and ethnic lines (Blackwelder, 1997). An important variable in the determination of professional behavior and how professions are regarded by others is education and, more specifically, the nature and type of educational institutions as well as the way knowledge is transferred. A source of debate in nursing, especially since the second half of the last century, is the amount, nature, and location of professional education. There has been a long and severe conflict internal to the profession over educational preparation for entry into practice.

Hospital-based nursing education programs historically have been the cornerstone of professional preparation. Known as diploma programs, they represent the oldest form of educational training leading to licensure as a professional nurse. At their foundation is a heavy emphasis on clinical experience and the skills needed to care for the acutely ill patient. These programs, originally based on the concept of apprentice education, reflected the model of the American family in that the roles of nurses and physicians were reminiscent of male and female roles in the family. Apprentice nurses heard of obedience and stringent discipline. They were docile and instilled with respect for authority and unswerving loyalty to the institution and physicians. In part, a lower status and less power for the nursing profession in comparison with other knowledge-based groups results from this apprentice-type nursing educational system dominated by the male model. Concentration on task-oriented courses has fueled a parochial outlook, discouraged participation in the larger community, and definitely not stimulated self-assertion (Bergman, 1985; Lowery-Palmer, 1982; Montgomery, 1994). It is interesting that, historically, critical thinking was not nurtured, even though Florence Nightingale, the founder of the nursing profession, based her activities on intelligence, thought and analysis. Moreover, in this original arrangement, combining service and education, service needs often took priority over the learning needs of students. Those who complete these hospital-based programs, which grant no college credit, receive a diploma. Graduates, not possessing an academic degree, encounter difficulties in continuing their education. For a wide variety of reasons that are beyond the scope of this work, diploma programs have experienced a severe decline in number. There has been a trend in nursing education away from these programs toward those in colleges and universities.

In the post World War II era a new approach to the preparation of nurses emerged that featured more flexible educational methods. As hospital programs became standardized in the late 1940s and early 1950s at the behest of the National League for Nursing, the organization responsible for all accrediting functions in the profession, many of them for educational and economic reasons, affiliated with an institution of higher education, principally a community college. Associate degree nursing programs, in which there is a required distribution between nursing and general education courses, first emerged in 1951 and it is these programs that have experienced the most growth. Their appearance brought about a change in the nursing student body, creating a more diverse group. However, Lynaugh and Brush (1996) observe: "Relocating nursing education from its traditional base in local hospital schools to mainstream educational institutions . . . acted to segment nursing, creating a caste system with discriminating racial and ethnic undertones" (p. 12). In fact today, as diploma programs have decreased in number, most minority graduates from basic nursing education programs possess the associate degree from a community college and most minority students currently enrolled in basic nursing education programs participate in associate degree programs. On the other hand, more than 41% of registered nurses hold a basic nursing or higher degree from a university (Keepnews, 1998; National Advisory Council on Nurse Education and Practice, 2000).

The identification of the professions with universities and institutions of higher education throughout the nineteenth and twentieth centuries demonstrates the relation of these groups to some branch of learning and science. The university has assumed a central and increasing importance to the total complex of professions. In the United States, professional training has been brought overwhelmingly within the university system and the nursing profession is no exception. Baccalaureate programs in nursing have existed since 1919. They provide the intellectual, cultural and technical components of a professional and liberal education. The course of study includes the liberal arts, science and humanities with a significant portion consisting of nonnursing courses. Focus is on the development of agents of change with critical decision-making judgments and elementary research skills. Universities have been important to professional evolution. In addition to furnishing social prestige,

> they can serve as legitimators, providing authoritative grounds for the exclusive exercise of expertise. They can house the function of knowledge advancement, enabling academic professionals to develop new techniques outside of practice. They can train young professionals, often in conjunction with the function of research. Finally, universities, like states, may become another arena for interprofessional competition. (Abbott, 1988, p. 196)

Thus, there are three types of basic educational paths that prepare individuals for licensure as a registered professional nurse: diploma, associate and baccalaureate programs. All feature diverse foci and outcomes. Yet products of these different arrangements take the same licensure examination, achieve the same title, fill the same positions, and even earn the same pay.

Since its birth, the ANA has been concerned with education. Debate on the issue of educational preparation intensified in the 1960s and especially in 1965 when its Committee on Education issued a position paper (American Nurses Association, 1965) on the subject, which was endorsed by the organization's governing body. Based on the notion that the education of health professionals must feature greater depth and breadth, baccalaureate programs were singled out for attention. The document affirmed: (1) Those desiring to become registered nurses should be prepared in institutions of higher education; (2) Entry to the ranks of professional nursing should require a baccalaureate degree; and (3) Technical nursing is based on associate degree preparation. These tenets, especially the emphasis on baccalaureate degree education, severely fragmented the profession and continue to do so. It is beyond the scope of this work to pursue the details and nuances of the schisms. Suffice it to say, they have gravely affected professional identity and unity.

In addition to a common expertise, professional identity is built on shared experiences and understandings as well as a common perception of problems and possible solutions. In part, this identity is created and re-created through generic professional training. Diverse educational routes have made the formation of a solidified and unified professional identity more difficult (Evetts, 1999). This lack of standardization of basic educational preparation has other consequences as well. One result is that these educational disparities often create an overproduction of practitioners and, thus, there is competition among professional nurses with different levels of training. Moreover, it has not allowed the profession to develop fully its potential strength. Given nursing's long history of education controlled by the hospitals, others were allowed to set standards for professional practice. If practitioners were powerless to establish their own tenets and guidelines, ". . . they could not perceive themselves as having power in relationship to other professionals within the health care system" (Lerner, 1985, pp. 90–91). These elements do not allow for the maturation of a pronounced assertive style in terms of communication and decision making. This past has influenced matters of rights and power.

The location of education, be it in the public or private sector, also impinges on professional behavior and institutions. Where educational institutions are in the public sector, such as in continental Europe, and especially Scandinavia, the nation-state and its agent, government, exercise control over the profession. On the other hand, in the United States professional education, not being embedded in the public sector and being privately organized, has, for the most part, created a presupposition that knowledge-based groups should be characterized by a negative attitude toward the state and its agent (Torstendahl, 1990).

THE WORK SETTING

The fact that most nurses work in bureaucratic settings also accounts for lack of empowerment and involvement in political activities. Moreover, patriarchy or generalized masculine domination pervades this environment. Gender, a principal determinant of social life, is the basis for the distribution of power and labor. Females, therefore, are subordinated to males and a masculine gender system prevails (Waters, 1989). Historically, nurses have been principally employed by hospitals, bureaucratic organizations mandating obedience to established policies and acceptance of orders, both of which reinforce the traditional socialization processes of nursing education. Most decisions have been made at the apex of the institutional structure and it has been expected that they would be implemented without question throughout the facility. Challenges by nursing staff members have been few and far between, given the possibility of job loss. In this environment nurses have been compliant and tractable subordinates to physicians and administrators. Hospitals and other health care institutions tend to be dominated by men and thus, male attitudes and male perspectives. In fact, the male-dominant, female-submissive social pattern reflected in the relations between nurses and physicians and nurses and hospital administrators has been perpetuated by institutional bureaucracies (Lewis, 1985).

The emphasis on rule-bound behavior has limited professional autonomy defined as ". . . the right of self-determination and governance without external control" (Kelly & Joel, 1996, p. 280). Successful professionalization is marked by achievement of autonomy, the single most important factor that characterizes a profession. It has two components: (1) autonomy of the character of the work or services being performed, meaning freedom to determine methods and procedures used, and (2) control over the context in which work is carried out, referring, among other things, to the establishment of territoriality, role relationships with other providers, and the cost of services. It is generally acknowledged that professionals must function autonomously in the development of professional policy and in the control of professional activity. Synonyms for freedom on the part of groups to dictate their own work behavior are self-regulation and self-control. Professions are distinguished from occupations on the basis of possession of this right to control their own work (McClelland, 1991; Pavalko, 1971; Rueschemeyer, 1993). This principle is reflected in federal legislation such as the Labor Relations Act of 1971 and its amendments. They affirm that a professional employee is one who, among other things, exercises discretion and judgment in performance of work responsibilities.

Laws regulating entry into the profession, established referral patterns, restrictions on certain forms of competition, exclusive professional competence in evaluating performance, and the presence of professional personnel in government are a few elements that ensure professional autonomy (Wilsford, 1991). In a discussion of this matter, Freidson (1973) cogently argues:

> Such power provides the framework for formal organization and control, the character for . . . license and mandate. It sets up the legal authority for the profession to recruit, train, examine, license and review performance, and establishes the formal limits of its exclusive jurisdiction. (p. 32)

Possession of professional sovereignty reaps many advantages. Among other things, it allows for control of supply and demand that, in turn, affords an opportunity for controlling prices, incomes and employment opportunities. American physicians exploited professional sovereignty to its fullest and, thus, became the arch of the health care delivery system. The profession has controlled medical education, the supply of providers and their incomes, among other elements. Nursing has not enjoyed this opportunity.

As noted, in the course of its development as a profession, nursing has been controlled by a variety of outside forces. Thus, it does not have the autonomy that is associated with the traditional notion of a profession. Individual practitioners as well as the profession as a whole experience restrictions on their autonomy. The precise amount of autonomy nurses possess depends on the specific employment site and the way in which work is organized. Public policy has limited nurses' professional autonomy by invoking three potent instruments: limitations on the scope of nursing practice, exclusionary definitions, and restrictions on eligibility for reimbursement. This mix of high skill and low autonomy and control is not unique to American nursing. The same pattern is a feature of the Canadian and British professions as well as others. It appears that the bureaucratic work context with its weak concern for autonomy is more palatable to females than to males. Having traditionally been more submissive than men, women have been more accepting of its authority. It might be asked if the scarcity of professional authority in nursing is due to the position of women in a patriarchal society (Leggatt, 1970; Walby & Greenwell, 1994).

REMUNERATION

It is generally acknowledged that women's work is not as highly valued in economic terms as the kinds of activities carried out by men or male-dominated professions. Gender is of considerable importance in the ranking of skills. Thus, no matter how skilled in a technical sense a profession might be, if it is a female one, it will rank low in terms of material rewards (Crompton, 1987). Nursing's inferior status is reflected in inadequate levels of compensation. Comparisons of nurses' earnings and working conditions with those of other professional and nonprofessional groups underscore their inferior economic position. For example, it has been shown that nurses have earned less than office, clerical and maintenance crew workers. The profession is also characterized by a serious salary compression. Over the span of a professional career, nurses can anticipate a salary increase of about 36%. Many reach this point five or six years after entering the workforce. This contrasts sharply with triple-digit-percentage increases for chemists, accountants, and computer programmers. Nor can nurses expect their wages to rise substantially as a result of longevity of service. Salaries for nurses are well below those for all female professionals, as well as those in male-dominated occupations requiring less skill and technical expertise. Furthermore, nurses are required to assume greater responsibility, necessitating more technical competence, without a concomitant increase in remuneration because of the salary compression problem. Due to a historic lack of wage competition, a "ratcheting" pay system developed that responds to cyclical supply-side nursing shortages with artificially low salaries (Friss,1988; Harrington, 1988; P. A. Kalisch & B. J. Kalisch, 1995; McCarthy, 1988). These harsh economic facts have been used to explain nursing's limited power. Economically, these professionals have not been able to take risks.

CULTURE AND SOCIALIZATION

Members of a profession have a common identity and a separate and distinctive subculture. Inherent in the preparation of the professional practitioner is the concept of occupational socialization, a complex process through which the individual becomes a professional being. It is concerned with the transmission of a network of information, feelings, norms, and beliefs that aid in actualizing a role and comprehending, evaluating and relating to a particular professional world and defining the relationship to the wider social structure. More specifically, as alluded to previously, this term is defined as the learning of norms, values, role behavior, orientations, self-conceptions, and ethical imperatives unique to a particular professional subculture as well as the specific skills and knowledge needed in the workplace. Professions tend to be more concerned with the nonskill elements of their cultures than the nonprofessions. Although students do not form cultural groups in the same sense as immigrants or primitives, in much the same way they are assimilated into a new realm, the professional world. Each professional constituency has a novel idea of the orientations its future members should possess. In short, via a complex socialization process, which varies according to profession, the future practitioner is molded to fit the needs of the profession and of society (Heinz, 1998; Olesen & Whittaker, 1970; Pavalko, 1971).

There are two general forms of professional socialization: direct and indirect. In the first, the nature of the substance transmitted is specifically professional. In the latter, the initial predispositions that are acquired are not necessarily professional, but they influence the subsequent development of specifically professional orientations. In other words, nonprofessional orientations are acquired first and then at a later date applied to the professional realm to create specific professional ones. There are various brands of direct and indirect socialization. Of particular importance to this study is anticipatory socialization of the direct variety. In this case people preparing for a profession often manifest the values and behavior associated with it long before they formally enter it. For example, nursing, law and medical students often begin to think and act like nurses, lawyers, and physicians long before they formally assume their professional roles. Future professionals, when they start their professional studies, bring with them diverse and varied conceptions and often misconceptions about the role to which they aspire and about the nature of the group to which they will belong. These notions depend on the individual's previous exposure to the profession. Often many of these orientations are changed to fit those of the profession. In the same vein, foreign-born nurses who have increased in number during periods of nursing shortages, are quickly socialized into the American profession.

Organizations that furnish a profession's pool of recruits and expand its fund of knowledge, principally educational institutions, are important components of the professional culture. In a statement referring to medical schools that is applicable to nursing programs, Merton (1957) commented:

> It is their function to transmit the culture of medicine and to advance that culture. It is their task to shape the novice into the effective practitioner of medicine, to give him the best available knowledge and skills, and to provide him with a professional identity so that he comes to think, act, and feel like a physician. It is their problem to enable the medical man to live up to the expectations of the professional role long after he has left the sustaining value-environment provided by the medical school. (p. 7)

One of the major purposes of the admissions process to professional schools is to identify and possibly eliminate individuals who are potentially strong deviants from the professional culture because of a deficiency in the appropriate values and motives for the anticipated roles, that, to a large extent, are learned in early life. Criteria other than academic qualifications are important. Thus, professions have been likened to social movements. Both recruit only certain types of people. They have their own specific ideologies and values in addition to their particular socialization mechanisms and both proselytize (Baim, 1972; Greenwood, 1972; Jackson, 1970).

Occupational socialization differs from other types in that, for the most part, it takes place in bureaucratic and, therefore, impersonal organizations, such as those institutions responsible for the education of the professional nurse. The type of educational programs in which they are enrolled, the basic philosophies of the associated health care institutions in which they practice and the personal values, philosophies, and behavior of their faculty members influence the socialization of nursing students. Institutions nurture excellence and allow students to use their abilities in the professional world. This experience is critical to the development of a professional self-concept. Obviously, professional socialization within this formal setting has a significant role in the explanation of individual behavior at the workplace, but by itself, it does not thoroughly explain it (Freidson, 1973). There are other aspects of the educational experience, other than the curriculum and the classroom, that are important in terms of socialization. Informal elements, such as contacts outside the formal classroom, the social climate, and extracurricular activities, to cite a few, must be considered along with the formal socialization agents. For example, the nature of the hospital hierarchy, and contacts with patients and other social elements, are important to this socialization process.

Socialization into the nursing profession may be divided into three phases. In the first the student develops a technical perspective of the occupation that replaces lay conceptions. Throughout the second phase that occurs in clinical training, ties with senior colleagues are developed and acceptance by them is based on professional criteria. They become significant others to the professional trainee. Finally, in the third phase, professional values are internalized, the profession becomes the dominant reference group and its expected behaviors are adopted. Faculty members become more important sources of professional behavior as the student progresses throughout the nursing program. Benchmark studies of professional socialization indicate that they become significant to the development of professional identity during the second clinical year and that students at the time of graduation manifest views and behavior similar to those of their faculty members (Dalme, 1983; Lynn, McCain, & Boss, 1989; Simpson, 1972).

Although not always successful, the final objective of occupational socialization is to produce orientations considered acceptable and proper by those who control the training and destiny of the students. Nursing faculty members are the most significant referents of behavior in terms of socialization into the profession. They command students' loyalty in the same way that the nursing principles stressed in training hold their interest. It is through faculty members that the classroom affects socialization. In addition to possessing authority in the classroom, faculty members enjoy a position of respect in society at large. Moreover, they provide an important source of values and attitudes about the profession. They are important to the professional socialization process because of the specific values, opinions and orientations that they hold, exhibit and disseminate. Like parents, they project their values and aspirations on their students. Furthermore, in the classroom they establish and manipulate a "learning culture" that, having important indirect consequences, can influence the outlook of the students.

Interaction with faculty members explains much of the students' professional behavior. Of special importance to participation in professional activities is faculty contact in informal settings. The more informal the student–faculty contact, the greater the influence the relationship has in the student's professional life. Student involvement in professional activities is related to the amount of contact with faculty members and the amount of encouragement received from them. Faculty members influence not only the amount of participation, but its nature as well. Contacts with these educators affect the students' view of the social and professional worlds. Such would suggest that important socialization processes are of the informal type (Pease, 1972). Faculty member influence is also important from another perspective. Nurse educators enjoy prestige and status as part of a professional elite that also includes the supervisors and nursing directors of large hospitals. Together they participate in the activities of an inner core of professional decision makers that controls the various professional associations and, therefore, sets the agenda for the rest of the constituency.

Although specific notions of a profession vary, it is generally recognized that one of its obligations is to reproduce its community. This reproduction is social in nature and is realized through the profession's control over entry to professional schools and the selection of new recruits who are socialized through training processes. Along with developing intellectual capacity as a decision maker, responsibility for patient welfare, and leadership potential, one of the talents that nursing programs, especially baccalaureate and higher-degree ones, endeavor to nurture in their students is participation in health care policy development. Nursing faculty members are responsible for effecting a sense of power not only within the nursing education system, but outside it as well. It is generally recognized that those in baccalaureate programs have the responsibility to familiarize students with health care policies and issues as well as to convey to them the notion that their involvement can make a difference (Batra, 1992; Goode, 1972). As will be noted throughout this work, these goals are not always achieved.

Given this mandate, occupational socialization includes a political facet and the development of the "political self." This notion refers to the individual's entire complex of orientations regarding the world of politics, including views of one's own political role. The core of the political self includes basic political sentiments, knowledge and evaluations of the structure and processes of politics and orientations toward more transient political objects such as policies, programs, personalities and events. Direct political socialization has a substantial impact on the development of the political self that is shaped by the interaction of three factors: the nature of the political system, the experiences and relationship the individual has with other individuals and groups, and the personal needs and capacities of the individual (Dawson, Prewitt, & Dawson, 1977).

Faculty role modeling of the knowledge, attitudes, and appropriate behaviors for impacting positively on the policy-making process is important to the development of political competence. Nurse educators in the classroom and outside it provide their students with models of various nursing roles. They are the most significant role models for fashioning the professional values and behavior of students and, thus, an important source for transmitting the professional subculture (Dalme, 1983). With role modeling, learning is based on observation. Behavioral patterns and social knowledge are acquired by observing the actions of specific esteemed figures who, serving as a point of reference, distribute "cultural capital" via their actions and appearance. In essence, socialization takes place through imitation. The desire to identify with professional colleagues and model one's comportment on theirs has a significant role in an individual's nursing socialization process. Often the person is converted in a religious sense, achieving a new self-identity and a new world view (Dubar, 1991; Zerwekh & Claborn, 1994). In these circumstances socialization is an active process. The motivation of the observer, the characteristics of the role model, the relationship between the former and the latter figures as well as the learning environment all determine the outcome (Bandura, 1977, 1986). Failure to model policy-related activities could lead incoming members of the profession to view these activities, although they are critical to them and their territoriality, as incongruous with the nursing role.

Socialization is a lifelong process throughout which changes in the forces to which the individual is exposed provide material for new social roles and a diverse self-identity. An important moment in the development of the political self is young adulthood, a period with multiple opportunities to participate in political activities. For the future professional nurse, an important part of this period occurs during formal professional education. Adult socialization is somewhat different from socialization that takes place in other phases of the life cycle. For the most part, it stresses overt behavior rather than motives and values (Baim, 1972; Heinz, 1998). This underscores the significance of nurse educators' role-modeling.

Obviously, what aspiring professionals learn in the course of their formal professional studies will have a major impact on their entire career. This is especially true in terms of socializing influence. Political learning has effects on the individual's political behavior at a later point in time and by extension on the profession and the political system. Socialization is a potential source of change (Greenstein, 1972). The seeds of change are present wherever and whenever different generations are exposed to diverse experiences and stimuli. The presence of these seeds is the key. Once present, professional forces and institutions must organize them and effectively channel them in the appropriate directions.

The factors presented in this chapter, among others, aid in an understanding of the functioning of the nursing profession, the way in which its members behave and the way in which it interacts with social and political structures. No one of these factors alone can be used as an explanatory variable. The professional fabric is revealed by the interplay of multiple elements, each or a combination, assuming a particular importance in specific circumstances. Having set forth some of these elements, we will now turn to a discussion of the survey and its relationship to the aforementioned themes.

Chapter 2

Nurse Educators: Who Are They and With Whom Do They Affiliate?

THE SURVEY: ITS NATURE

It has been established that nurse educators are essential to the socialization process and the continuous development of the nursing profession. The questionnaire was administered to faculty members in baccalaureate and higher degree programs in New York State for two principal reasons. As noted earlier, the entry into practice issue has long divided the profession. At the 1995 meeting of the governing and official voting body of the ANA, the House of Delegates, consisting of elected representatives from the ANA's constituent associations and the Board of Directors, this matter once again served as a source of debate. On this occasion 80% of the delegates supported the position that a baccalaureate degree in nursing be required for entry into professional practice. More recently, at meetings in 2000 and 2001, the association's board of directors reaffirmed its long-standing commitment to this orientation. In light of such decisions, baccalaureate and higher-degree programs were selected for this study. It is expected that entry into practice in the near future will require a baccalaureate degree. Obviously, the consistent reaffirmation of such a policy enhances the prominence of a major component of the professional elite, nursing faculty in colleges and universities. This group is important because as Abbott (1988) has written:

> Academic knowledge legitimizes professional work by clar-ifying its foundations, tracing them to major cultural values. In most modern professions, these have been the values of rationality, logic and science. Academic professionals demonstrate the rigor, the clarity, and the scientifically logi-cal character of professional work, thereby legitimating that work in the context of larger values. (p. 54)

Also, surveys of nursing programs reveal that the largest in-crease in enrollments in the past has been experienced by baccalau-reate programs. However, according to the American Association of Colleges of Nursing, enrollments of entry-level bachelor's degree stu-dents in the nation's nursing schools fell by 2.1% in 2000, the sixth consecutive decline in as many years. Still, in terms of their faculty and students, baccalaureate programs are of great importance to the nursing profession. Reduced enrollments in all types of entry-level nursing programs are attributed to a number of factors, including a shortage of faculty in these programs, a redirection of limited re-sources to meet the demand for advanced practice nurses, and a fail-ure on the part of potential students to understand the new demand for nursing personnel and changed and changing career opportuni-ties. Unfortunately, there are no recent data available concerning en-rollment in nursing programs in New York State. The regular collection of general data on the nursing profession is not mandated ("ANA at Work," 1999; Brewer & Kovner, 2000; Freudenheim & Villarosa, 2001).

New York State was selected as a research site because it occu-pies a special place in the history of nursing. Many of the profession's visionary leaders, such as Lillian Wald, Lavinia Dock, Margaret Sanger, Ruth Watson Lubic and Eleanor Lambertsen, were active in that state's professional nursing organization, the New York State Nurses Association. Being externalists, they not only left their mark on the state, but the impact of their activities went far beyond and ex-tended to the nation. These women provided role modeling in politi-cal activism that became an ideal for some members of the nursing elite. Moreover, New York State has achieved several "firsts." The first state nurses' association in the United States was formed there. In addition, this organization initiated the principal statutory movements in nursing's early professionalization endeavors. More recently, in 1971, a group of nurses from New York State, realizing that nursing had no internal structure with which to influence different points of the political arena, formalized the drive for involvement in the political system. They formed a nonpartisan, nonprofit association of registered and practical nurses called Nurses for Political Action. This organization was the forerunner to the American Nurses Association's Political Action Committee.

Moreover, in 1973 the New York State Nurses Association was a significant force in the passage of a revised nurse practice act. This legislation acknowledged nursing as an autonomous profession. It differentiated nursing and medical practice and set forth nurses' independent functions. Nursing was defined as "diagnosing and treating human responses to actual or potential health problems through such means as case finding, health teaching, and counseling" (P. A. Kalisch & B. J. Kalisch, 1995, p. 452). With this definition the practice of nursing for the first time could claim a statutory authority. A year later the New York State Nurses Association came to grips with the entry-into-practice issue. It was the first state nurses association to pass a resolution mandating the baccalaureate degree as the minimum requirement for entry into professional practice. Such action quickly became a part of the national professional nursing agenda (V. L. Bullough & B. Bullough, 1984; Driscoll, 1994; Hall-Long, 1995b; Mason & Leavitt, 1995; Rothberg, 1985). Of all the state nursing associations, the one in New York State has established a reputation as a prime mover and shaker.

The data on which the ensuing discussion is based stem from the aforementioned survey administered in spring 1996 by mail. The questionnaire consisted of open- and close-ended questions designed to elicit data relating to (1) membership and level of participation in professional and other policy-related organizations; (2) electoral behavior; (3) knowledge of, position on, and participation in policy development related to key national and state issues affecting nursing; (4) opinions concerning factors affecting the type and level of participation in policy development by professionals; (5) knowledge of, access to, and use of nursing literature concerned with public policy; (6)

opinions on nursing, the profession, its status, and policy development and (7) demographics. The sampling frame included the 418 full-time nursing faculties in 25 baccalaureate and higher-degree programs in New York State. Prior to its administration, the survey instrument was subjected to a pretest. The response rate was 60% with 250 useable questionnaires returned.

THE RESPONDENTS: A PROFILE

Given that nursing is among the most sharply sex-segregated of professions (95% female), and primarily a white one (89%), as might be expected, respondents were predominately female (98%) and white (93%). In terms of gender and ethnic/racial background, the sample closely resembled the general profile of American nurse educators in which male faculty account for three percent of the group and racial/ethnic minorities represent nine percent. Not only are minorities seriously underrepresented in the ranks of nurse educators, but the same holds true in terms of their representation in the general nursing and other health professions nationwide and in New York State. Moreover, the percentage of minority nurses still lags behind the percentage of minorities within the general population. Racial/ethnic minority groups comprise 28% of the American population and less than 10% of all registered nurses. This underrepresentation promises to become more severe in the near future. The percentage of minority nurses has tended to remain stable, while it is predicted that racial/ethnic minorities will account for 40% of the United States' population by 2020. Although there is a high concentration of minorities in New York State (36%), a significant majority of registered nurses employed in nursing (77%) are white (Bureau of Health Professions, 2000a, 2000b; National Advisory Council on Nurse Education and Practice, 2000; National League for Nursing, 1995; Rosella, Regan-Kubinski, & Albrecht, 1994; Sower, 1996). Racial exclusion and gender stratification mark American nursing.

For African Americans, the profession developed slowly. The first African American nurse was graduated in 1879 and by the start of the last century there were many black nurses. However, they con-

fronted discrimination, by law in the S
North (Carnegie, 1994). Facing exclusi
in the ANA, these service providers ha
National Association of Colored Grad
fierce and sustained attack against di
the profession. However, it was onl
with the ANA.

Although male nurses have existed an.
nurses in the United States, they experienced and su..
ficulty in the profession. Reflecting Florence Nightingale's be.
to be a "good nurse" was also to be a "good woman," nursing be
came almost exclusively a feminized occupation during the late nineteenth century. American nursing fashioned by the stamp of Florence
Nightingale had no meaningful place for men. An exception was the
case in which physical strength was needed. Thus, males were used to
care for alcoholics, and mentally ill and violent patients. Also because
of the prevailing belief that intimate contact with strange men was inappropriate for young unmarried women, they were used to treat
men with genitourinary diseases. Originally, nurse training schools
were only open to females. A decade and a half after the founding of
the first schools of nursing, the training of male nurses for general patient care became a possibility in 1888. However, opportunities were
not initially widespread and it is only in the late twentieth century
that men have increasingly found their way back to nursing (Brown
et al., 2000).

Like African Americans in the profession, male nurses suffered
discrimination. For them the situation was similar to that of women
working in a male-dominated field. Not all of the prejudicial treatment was the fault of nursing. Other forces, such as sentiment, role
stereotyping, and tradition were involved. The link between women
and nursing was and still is a strong one. The work of nursing and
the nurse in the public mind are affiliated with females. The qualities
of care, concern, responsibility, nurturance, gentleness, empathy,
compassion, tenderness, unselfishness, comfort and understanding,
among others, are frequently assumed to be feminine virtues. A
woman doing nursing is usually described as a "nurse," whereas a
male doing the same work will often be referred to as a "male nurse"
(Davies, 1995). World War II provides another example. This conflict
enhanced opportunities for African American nurses, but it militated

in the profession. The cause of the former was em-
_ National Housing Council for War Service, the White
_ Eleanor Roosevelt. On the other hand, no strong move-
_ fair treatment for men wanting a nursing education and
_ntering military service was ever seriously launched. The pre-
_ng view within the establishment, most of the nursing profession,
_d the public was that men belonged on the battlefield and nursing
was women's work. Consequently, male nurses were kept in the regular armed services until 1966 when, as a result of professional pressure, they were allotted places in the Nurse Corps. The title of a book
chapter (Roberts & Group, 1995) aptly describes this situation: "The
Paradox: Nurses as Healers in Men's Horrible Wars." Much of the
discrimination that male nurses have had to face results from this
larger societal gender bias (Burtt, 1998). The reversal of this feminine
stereotyping of nurses requires a massive resocialization of the general public. The process has been slow and still continues. Even
though the psychological restraining forces identified with femininity
are still evident, B. Bullough (1983) observes that with more men in
the profession, nurses became more assertive.

Racial and gender stratification has increased as nurses pursue
advanced education. Minority health-care providers in general, and
nurses in particular, are important to an improvement in the health
status of today's minority or emerging majority. With the scope of
achieving an equitable representation of the diversity in American society within the ranks of nursing and its elite, recruitment efforts were
intensified and nursing workforce diversity programs bloomed. The
harvest has not met expectations. Reasons for its lesser yield include
lack of role models, lack of understanding of the true nature of the
profession, lack of proper counseling and an inability to meet standards due to poor academic records (Kelly & Joel, 1996; Rosella et
al., 1994). New strategies to enhance recruitment and innovative support systems must be devised.

In spite of these enhanced recruitment efforts aimed at racial minority groups and men, the situation reflected in this sample currently
prevails. The underrepresentation of minorities among nurse educators only perpetuates underrepresentation of minorities in the nursing
student body and workforce. This, in turn, has severe implications
for the delivery of culturally sensitive health care. Moreover, it has
long been recognized that the social composition of a teaching staff

impinges on the views students manifest toward various social and political phenomena. Thus, this noticeable absence of minority presence among the nursing leadership strata in general, and nurse educators in particular, is of special concern as diversity continues to grow in American society.

Respondents to the survey may be labeled "middle-aged." Seventy-six percent were between the ages of 40 and 59 with a roughly even distribution at either end of the age continuum—that is, in the 30–39 and the 60-and-over categories. Surprisingly, no participant was under 30. This compares with a 1996 national nursing sample survey that indicated that the average age of registered nurses was 44.3 years and later data issued by the Bureau of Health Professions showing an average age of 45.2 and rising (Freudenheim & Villarosa, 2001; "New Nursing Data," 1997). According to a 1999 survey of 535 of the nation's nursing schools by the American Association of Colleges of Nursing, the average age of full-time nursing faculty members was 50. In New York State a survey of registered nurses in 1995 revealed that the population of nurses had considerably advanced in age following national trends and a year later the Bureau of Health Professions confirmed this fact, noting that in this particular Census Division the registered nurse workforce aged considerably. The percentage of practitioners 40 years of age and older had risen to 63% (Bureau of Health Professions, 2000a; Sower, 1996). This aging pattern seems to be more developed in this sample. In either case, the mean age of the population indicates that there is really a very small youthful group of nurses. The dearth of nurse educators under 30 years of age in the sample reflects the dramatic decrease in the proportion of the registered nurse workforce younger than 30 years (Buerhaus, Staiger, & Auerbach, 2000). Nurse educators in baccalaureate and higher-degree programs, like New York State nurses, are aging. Sixty-five percent of the sample was married and 18%, 13% and three percent represented single, divorced/separated, or widow/widower status respectively.

As far as basic nursing preparation is concerned, a majority (53%) of respondents held a baccalaureate degree and 25% a diploma. Ten percent had an associate degree, four percent a doctorate in nursing science and the rest had either a combination of diploma/baccalaureate or associate degree/baccalaureate. The sample differs from its national counterpart in terms of highest earned credential. Nationally, 45% of full-time nurse faculty held a doctorate (National League for Nursing, 1995) and in the New York State sample, the percentage was 54. Although the percentage of those holding a doctorate was higher in the case of New York State, when compared with the academic credentials of other university departments, it is quite low. In the academy, a basic requirement for a faculty appointment, tenure, and promotion is a doctoral degree in one's field of specialization. This creates a problem of status for nurse educators, many of whom do not have a doctorate or if they do, frequently it is in a field other than nursing. In fact, many nurse educators have advanced degrees in education. The doctorate in nursing is a relatively new degree. It was only in the 1960s that graduate education in nursing, especially at the master's level, began to flourish. In the next decade, increased emphasis on doctoral education became evident. However, in both cases graduate-level content in nursing was not extensively developed. Many programs initially stressed nonnursing areas, such as administration or teaching. Moreover, nurse educators do not always adhere to the generally acknowledged basic credential and tenure standards in terms of education, scholarly endeavors, research and teaching. Although nursing is a discipline in the sciences and a practice-oriented profession, nursing faculty members who engage in clinical experiences often encounter obstacles in their bids for promotion and tenure. Formal policies for advancement in the academy clash with practice mandates of the profession.

Nurse educators frequently, in spite of a lack of scholarly productivity, progress throughout an academic career. The justification for such a practice is the lack of nurses with doctoral degrees and a research agenda and, thus, the need to use lesser qualified individuals. This situation jeopardizes the very foundation of nursing education (P. A. Kalisch & B. J. Kalisch, 1995). Very often these educators carry heavier teaching loads than colleagues in other departments and they, therefore, have less time for research endeavors. It is a vicious cycle. Also, the heavy emphasis on research in many academic institutions detracts from the importance of clinical work. One analysis of nursing faculty workload found that less time was given to research than any other activity and that only a half of the respondents spent any time at all in research-related activities (Solomons, Jordison, & Powell, 1980).

As might be expected, with the expansion of graduate education, nursing research experienced growth. Not only has individual nursing research increased, but there is an apparent augment in non-nursing research as well (Kinsey, 1986). A more recent survey involving New York State nurse educators (Smolowitz & Murray, 1997) reports an increase in the quality and quantity of research that focuses primarily on clinical evaluation and educational studies. Of significance to the policy endeavors of the nursing profession is that only one work related to health care policy. This phenomenon reflects the fact that relatively few nursing publications are classified as primarily policy research. Articles recently published in the principal professional nursing journals concern clinical research, methodological issues, and the applied sciences. Although there has been an increase in the number of articles relying on qualitative methods, quantitative approaches dominate the field. Research on nursing's political socialization is still in its infancy. There is a dearth of nursing policy research in nursing and nursing policy analysis research by nurses. These areas require further development (M. E. Evans, 1995; Hall-Long, 1995b).

One shortcoming of nursing's research efforts is that they have not had a significant impact on public policy. For the most part, the implications of findings are not projected beyond professional practice to the public policy arena. Moreover, the noncumulative nature of nursing research, its insufficient replication, and its restricted dissemination limit its impact on public policy. An exception to this state of affairs has been provided by the public policy studies undertaken by nurse-midwives. The success of these endeavors is explained by their simplicity, their presentation, and their style, which are easy to understand, and their focus on issues of concern to policy makers (Milio, 1989; Raudonis & Griffith, 1991).

The fact that many nurse educators have advanced degrees in education has impacted negatively on their research efforts. Their graduate training in the immediate past did not contain the research component identified with other doctoral programs. It emphasized curriculum, supervision, social foundations, educational psychology and similar fields all of which might be relevant to nursing. However, it did not stress specific nursing problems or research techniques. To a large degree, this preparation focused on how to teach nursing, rather than on the individual scientific or scholarly inquiry affiliated with the various disciplines. As a result, nurse educators, instead of carrying out research on topics affecting nursing often opted to study and implement curriculum revision. V. L. Bullough and B. Bullough (1984) observe: "Not infrequently, the result was a kind of ghetto mentality in which nurses tended to find the solution in curriculum revision" (p. 45). This was natural, given the nature of their graduate program. Education was stigmatized by the other disciplines and by identifying with it, nursing was stigmatized as well.

After World War II, extensive changes took place in the American health care system, generating a modified role for health care professionals and fertile ground in which to sow the seeds of research. Nursing lagged behind in terms of the challenge. The generation of new knowledge for the profession was not synchronized with society's health needs (P. A. Kalisch & B. J. Kalisch, 1995). In 1950 the ANA House of Delegates launched a major research program for the interdisciplinary study of nursing functions in diverse settings and geographic areas as well as relationships between nurses and their colleagues on the health care team. Much of the effort was initially undertaken by social scientists, but eventually nurses, obtaining the requisite skills, became more involved. At the same time, a professional journal, appropriately entitled *Nursing Research*, came into being to disseminate scholarly output.

Inquiry was further energized by the extramural grants program in nursing research of the United States Public Health Service Division of Nursing Resources. From 1956 on, this program supported individual research efforts, faculty research development projects, and several special national nursing research conferences held under the auspices of the ANA. The creation of the National Center for Nursing Research (NCNR) in 1986, in spite of a presidential veto and opposition from the powerful National Institutes of Health, was a milestone in the history of the profession. Its significance derived from the fact that it symbolized the value of nursing research. It was established

> for the purpose of conducting a program of grants and awards supporting nursing research and research training related to patient care, the promotion of health, the prevention of disease, and the mitigation of the effects of acute

and chronic illness and disabilities. In support of studies on nursing interventions, procedures, delivery methods and ethics of patient care the NCNR programs are expected to complement other biomedical research programs that are primarily concerned with the causes and treatment of disease. (cited in Kelly & Joel, 1996, pp. 214–215)

Six years after its birth the center achieved the full status of an institute when it became the National Institute for Nursing Research. Nursing had come of age in terms of research. The Institute supports research, research training, and career development in health promotion and disease prevention, acute and chronic illness, and nursing systems. Research priorities are selected on an annual basis.

In the United States, nursing research has generally progressed through three stages: the establishment of university-based nursing programs, the introduction of research-based education in the form of master's programs aimed at research utilization in the nursing sector, and the creation of Ph.D. programs to prepare specialized researchers in the field (Elzinga, 1990). All of the aforementioned developments related to the institutionalization of research efforts are commendable because the amount of monies available to nurses has always been substantially less than that accessible to the other health care professions. In addition, nurses' research efforts have been hindered because they compete with physicians for access to subjects and many nurses are not aware of the importance of research to their practice. The late development of nursing research has borne severe consequences for the development of the profession's knowledge base and it has delayed professionalization.

Research is another issue that has divided the ranks of nursing. There are differing views concerning its purpose and direction. One camp views it as a means to a political end—in this case, respect and position in the academic world—that it hopes will spill over to other arenas. Another school believes that research produces answers to questions that guide knowledge-based nursing practice in clinical, educational and administrative roles. Although both parties accept that all research endeavors enhance nursing's status, there is tension between them about the purpose of various research undertakings. Baer (1987) traces these differences to the culture of nursing. She writes: ". . . Nursing's long history of keeping order and following procedure manuals restricted its ability to accept the multiple dimensions of ideas that often characterize educated thinking" (p. 19).

A matter for debate is the relationship between teaching, research, and clinical practice. Sherwin (1998) asks if a faculty member in a professional discipline, such as nursing, is a scholar and competent to teach without engaging in some form of practice. She argues for a change in policies to make possible not only support for faculty who engage in clinical undertakings, but reward. Moreover, the Pew Health Professions Commission (1993) claims that excellence in clinical care and service should be recognized in the tenure and promotion system. Evaluation of the nurse educator's productivity presents a challenge, given the ascriptive values of the academy (Ruby, 1998).

Higher education as well as the creation of linkages with and inroads into research are important for professionalization. In attempting to gain autonomy and status by moving out of the context of hospital settings and into the educational mainstream, nurse educators immediately became engaged in another struggle—that of gaining respectability in the halls of academe. In the academy there is a relationship between power and prestige. Empirical studies have shown that departments that rank high in academic prestige also rank high in power. Nursing is not included in this category. Often, not possessing the minimal academic credential, failing sometimes to meet the basic criteria for tenure and promotion, and being part of a female profession, nurse educators encounter a lack of respect and severe criticism from colleagues in other disciplines. Lack of status in the university community has been linked to a lack of status in the occupational structure. Although it might enjoy a favorable public image, the status of the nursing profession in terms of salary, working conditions and level of autonomy is not especially high. This reflects back on the academic standing of nursing faculties that operate under another disadvantage, that of being a relatively recent arrival on the academic scene, accounting for their lack of fully established currency. Thus, nurse educators are sometimes placed outside the mainstream of university life and, for all practical purposes, relegated to second-class citizenship. In encounters with scholars from other disciplines, they are not among equals. Often the power position of nurse educators is reflected in their lack of control of nursing educational programs. Of note is that, as opposed to their counterparts in other fields, some nursing deans have had less control over their resources. More specifically, they have not really controlled their budgets nor have they had authority over capitation and other nursing monies (Becher, 1990; V. L. Bullough & B. Bullough, 1984; Levi, 1980; Solomons et al., 1980; Williamson, 1983). This is another illustration of the fact that in the course of its development as a profession, nursing has been controlled by a variety of outside forces.

Sixty-seven percent of the participants in the survey held a master's degree in nursing and six percent obtained this degree in another field. In their graduate education, respondents pursued a wide variety of clinical and functional areas. Most prominent are psychiatric/mental health, public health, community, medical/surgical, and adult nursing; education, research and administration. Forty-four percent of the sample was certified in an area of specialty practice by a national certifying body. As might be expected, this percentage is considerably higher than the national one for registered nurses (6%) ("New Nursing Data," 1997).

In terms of employment, 55% of the sample was affiliated with a nursing program granting baccalaureate and higher degrees. In this category the distribution between the public and private sectors was almost equal. Thirty-one percent taught in either public or private baccalaureate programs. Those teaching in nursing programs affiliated with religious institutions represented the smallest part of the sample—14%.

Junior faculty (lecturer, instructor, assistant professor) accounted for 48% of the sample and 13% were clinical faculty members. Thirty-six percent were senior faculty (associate professor or higher) and the small percentage remaining had disparate titles. More specifically, 32% were assistant professors and 23% associate professors. This picture differs from the national one in which the former accounts for 42% of full-time baccalaureate and higher-degree faculty and the latter accounts for 27%. Also, there is a slight lack of congruence in the figures for professors in the sample and on a national basis. In general, nationally, less than 10% of full-time faculty hold the rank of professor (National League for Nursing, 1995). In the sample, 13% fell in this category.

Given the age distribution of the respondents, it is surprising that most of them (60%) were untenured. This fact might temper in the New York State case the previously discussed practices in the nursing academy. Faculty salary for six percent of the respondents was under $30,000, with three percent earning less than $20,000. Those earning between $30,000 and $40,000 and between $40,000 and $50,000 accounted for the largest number of participants (32%). Twenty-four percent earned between $50,000 and $60,000 and 13% had a salary of $60,000 or over. As often happens with survey research, many (one-quarter of the sample) did not reply to the question concerned with income.

To understand demands on their time in addition to their academic responsibilities, participants in the survey were asked if they engaged in other professional activities, such as private practice, consultation, and so on. Seventy-five percent of the sample responded in the affirmative. The primary reasons given for such activities in order of their importance were: continued professional development, provide additional income to supplement my faculty salary, and maintain/enhance my clinical skills. The last two mentioned motives received equal response rates. Obviously, these other activities impinge on research efforts.

In an attempt to obtain a fuller picture of their involvement outside academia, respondents were asked about their memberships in organizations related to the community at large, such as the League of Women Voters, Democratic and Republican clubs, or those of an independent nature. These secondary groups act as socialization agents, although they vary in terms of their political environment and the amount of influence they exert over their members and others. They engage in direct and indirect socialization. Moreover, they provide a framework for the development of primary relationships that impact on political orientations and a point of reference for individual decision making. In terms of the political socialization process, these groups are important because they help develop leadership talents and offer experiences and training in group relations. In all cases, the nonmembership category applied to well over 90% of the sample and in those cases in which membership was held, active membership, meaning "regularly attend program meetings," and so on, was minuscule, hovering at about one percent.

Certain common patterns concerning the political identification of health care professionals have been established. Representing elite and gratified sectors in society, they are, more often than not, con-

servative rather than liberal in their political orientations (Vollmer &
Mills, 1966). Participants in this survey did not mirror this general
tendency. A majority (52%) thought of themselves as Democrats and
22% indicated a propensity for the Republican Party. Fifteen percent
opted for an independent identity. Four percent thought of themselves as something else and six percent had no preference. Republicans and Democrats differed on the intensity of their political party
affiliation. Only eight percent claimed to be strong Republicans,
whereas the percentage for strong Democrats was 36.Thus, Democrats had a stronger bond with their political party. Nationwide surveys of members of state nurses associations second the Democratic
and liberal political leaning of the sample. In these polls more members favored the Democratic Party and they were more Democratic
and liberal than the general public ("ANA Takes Poll," 1996; de-
Vries, 1996).

PROFESSIONAL NURSING ORGANIZATIONAL AFFILIATIONS

Every profession operates through a network of formal groups
that includes professional associations. For some scholars (Carr-Saunders & Wilson, 1933), part of the professional development process
involves the establishment of such an organization. Powerful instruments that play a prominent role in empowering individuals in their
emerging professionalism, these groups are important in terms of the
establishment of professional norms, identity, and solidarity, as well as
education and information exchange. The opinions and values of people tend to be created, sustained, and altered by the groups and asso-
ciational ties of which they are a part. Having a political dimension,
these secondary groups operate concurrently as political socialization
forces. In fact, they perform strategic roles in the socialization process.
Also, they are themselves socialized by their participation in public affairs. They provide structural supports for political participation and
act as bearers of ideas. They serve as a framework for collaboration
and as initiators and reinforcers of political behavior as well as a point
of reference for political and professional decision making. They serve
the useful function of articulating the self-image and wishes of the
members of the profession. In addition to nurturing a commitment to

values and norms central to the tasks of the profession, they influence the content and structure of the "political self." The structure and culture of the profession further institutionalize these values and norms. Through membership in professional organizations, individuals are afforded an opportunity to be a part of the collective professional voice and to develop and enhance political skills (J. Greenwood, 1997; Hanley, 1987; Rains, 1988; Vollmer & Mills, 1966; Zerwekh & Claborn, 1994).

Lavinia Dock, one of nursing's rebellious advocates, vigorously underscored the significance of professional associations by arguing that they were really the true schools for general education. Their importance stemmed from their transmission of ethics and their role in refining perceptions and providing opportunities to form judgments. Consequently, in her eyes, they were institutions of lifelong learning (James, 1985). They are significant because

> [F]ormal programs provide training for younger members. Officers and members learn about human relations, public speaking and organizational skills. And many members exchange information and tricks of the trade in informal conversation . . . before and after meetings. The associational aim of maintaining occupational competence is not only promoted through formal education and informal socialization, there is also the process of certification, [and] the control of entry . . . functions often delegated . . . by the government to professional associations. . . . [Moreover,] some occupational associations openly operate as direct pressure groups in the formation of public policy. . . . (Strauss, 1963, p. 21 cited, in Vollmer & Mills, 1966, p. 161)

In spite of their noted importance to knowledge-based groups, it is noteworthy that Florence Nightingale did not recognize the need for professional associations which were not as well developed in her time as they are today. For her, the core of nursing resided in the individual. However, given these varied functions, professionals draw heavily on their professional associations as a reference group, like the family, churches, and other organizations, for guidance on attitudes and issues.

The American Nurses Association

A fact lamented in the nursing literature is that in spite of its importance, most nurses do not belong to the ANA, the official voice of nursing and the only full-service professional nursing organization. It is generally acknowledged that only about 10% of the total nursing population has held membership in the association (B. Bullough & V. L. Bullough, 1994; Joel, 1985; Schutzenhofer & Musser, 1994). This has been a long-standing trend. Although there has been an increase in the number of nurses, ANA membership has remained relatively stable for the past fifty years and has recently decreased to about seven percent of the profession. In fact, total membership is the same as it was twenty years ago (American Nurses Association, 2001). Findings in this study second the notion that many nurses are not affiliated with the official voice of nursing. In terms of this sample, the incidence of membership was much higher than that for the nation. Twenty percent of the respondents claimed they were active members. Of these, 18% were local or state leaders and one percent provided national leadership. This finding supports the notion that those who do participate in the association are frequently the leaders in the profession. It is noteworthy that only one percent of the active members was not included in the leadership strata. The role of nurse educators in the nursing elite is confirmed. These people share some, but not all, of the characteristics of a "typical" ANA member who is female, white, between 35 and 49 with an associate or baccalaureate degree in nursing, works full time in a hospital as a staff nurse, has been in this position for at least five years and in the field of nursing for twenty or more years, and has a total family income of more than $50,000 (deVries, 1996). On the other hand, 61% of this sample were nonmembers (28%) or inactive members (33%), in the latter case meaning they only contributed to the treasury of the organization and provided a name for the roll.

The realities of respondents' membership in the official professional organization are interesting when examined in light of their beliefs concerning such membership. Seventy percent of the sample supported the notion that all nursing faculty members should be active members of the official professional association. Only 16% dissented. Twelve percent was undecided and two percent had no opinion. In addition, an overwhelming majority (95%) affirmed that nursing students should be socialized into valuing membership and being active in the professional association. The respondents' actions are not congruent with their beliefs. Obviously, there is a significant difference between theory and practice. The behavior of participants in this regard demonstrates that they fail to understand the implications of being group oriented. This same trend will be identified in their responses to other items on the questionnaire. Nursing faculty in baccalaureate and higher-degree programs in New York State reflect the apathy and lack of interest of their nursing colleagues across the nation as it relates to the official voice of nursing. This is significant because the respondents' state affiliate, the New York State Nurses Association, as noted previously, is the oldest and among the most active in the nation. Other state associations view it as a leader.

In the early 1950s, belonging to a professional nursing organization was in vogue. However, within three decades membership in the ANA declined by 10 to 15%, while the number of nurses increased by 150%. Prior to the decline, membership had remained relatively stable despite an increase in the nurse population. Membership in professional nursing organizations has been researched by many and there have been no conclusive findings of how or why nurses select nursing associations (Lowery-Palmer, 1982; Zerwekh & Claborn, 1994). In any case, it is obvious that nursing's socialization process has fallen short in conveying the important implications of being group oriented. Certainly members of the profession in general and, in particular, respondents to this survey, have not heeded the words of Lavinia Dock, who at the dawn of the century argued: ". . . There is no teacher like voluntary association, no means of developing character greater than that offered by associated life . . ."(James, 1985, p. 44).

Any voluntary organization to attract members must see to it that the benefits of membership outweigh the financial costs. In the case of the state nurses' associations, various reasons have been advanced for their failure to achieve this objective. Typical is the statement that "we see little benefit from our membership . . ." ("Membership Matters," 1995) and a continuing source of irritation to many nurses is the high cost of annual dues. Also, there has not been universal support within the nursing community for all the activities of the professional organization. For example, some of the services, such as collective bargaining, are controversial. For a segment of the nursing community it is incompatible with professionalism. Lack of agreement with the policy orientations of the organization and the scope of its policy agenda also explains why many nurses fail to join their major professional association. There is a variety of opinion related to the issues with which a professional association should be concerned.

The ANA has been further weakened by the fact that many nurses did and do not view nursing as a career, but rather as an occupation. This tendency also impinges negatively on the development of a professional culture at the heart of which lies the career concept. This means that work should not be viewed solely as a means to an end, as has often been the case in nursing, but as the end itself. Noting that curing the ill is a value in itself, Ernest Greenwood (1972) writes: "The professional performs . . . services primarily for the psychic satisfactions and secondarily for the monetary compensations . . ." (pp. 13–14). For many clinicians, nursing is not perceived as a career and, thus, nurse employment has varied according to the life cycle of the nurse who very often worked until marriage and then left the ranks of the world of work to raise a family. After children had grown, some returned to the fold and some did not. Moreover, nurses did not perceive themselves as the primary wage earners in the family. Their income was viewed as a supplement to that of their spouse and employment was generally sought in the locale where a spouse had work. Membership in the major professional association was not important to one's career or to the ability to find a job. Thus, under these conditions the economic benefits of affiliating with the group were open to question. The financial costs definitely exceeded the advantages (Feldstein, 1988; Hriceniak, 1994; B. J. Kalisch & P. A. Kalisch, 1976; Orsolits et al., 1983). Even if some of these people did belong to the professional organization at one point in their career, say before marrying and their exit to raise a family, this turnover in membership from the perspective of the professional interest group is damaging. It is a debilitating factor that obstructs the creation of an important political resource, a cohesive, active membership base.

Time pressures also serve as another reason for not assuming a commitment. Given the responsibilities of work and home, many nurses feel that they cannot afford the time required for participation. Closely related is the argument that meetings are too distant from one's place of work or residence. Also, competition from other organizations within nursing and outside must be considered as well. One only has so much time to devote to voluntary associations. The costs and benefits for membership in each one must be calculated and prioritized. It might be that the major nursing organization does not adequately address the welfare of its constituency and membership is being sought elsewhere. The attitude toward affiliating with the ANA for many who fail to do so may be summed up with a typical comment on the subject: "[I]t doesn't do anything for you." Lowery-Palmer (1982) notes:

> Implied in this response is the traditional view of self that leads nurses to look to others to make decisions and take actions for them. Such a view of self accounts in large measure for the traditional reluctance of nurses to unite and fight for their personal and professional interest. (p. 195)

Even though the professional association is the single most powerful mechanism available to nurses, given this attitude and the low level of membership, it is difficult for the ANA to speak effectively for the nursing profession. It has a tradition of representing nurses on issues related to their profession, but this tradition is at risk. In the words of Lucille Joel (1985), a former president of the association:

> The ANA will only speak for nursing as long as it represents more nurses than any other organization. Our representativeness is already being challenged. It becomes difficult to influence public policy and cultivate political alliances when the organization can no longer claim to speak for large numbers of individuals and consequently the profession. (p. 105)

This affirmation is still valid today. Its low membership figures demonstrate that the ANA has much to do before it can confidently claim to represent the nursing profession. It must provide sufficient incentives so that membership becomes a valuable commodity and it must reconsider the nature of the constituency's common interests. Are they economic? Are they related only to nursing? Are they concerned with broader issues? With its Membership Project Management Team and its Futures Task Force, the ANA is addressing these matters and more in search of answers.

At one time it was thought that common needs and group consciousness were all that was necessary for group formation and effectiveness in the political arena. However, this thesis was harshly challenged in a stellar study by Mancur Olson (1965), who illustrated that organizing and maintaining an interest group is not an easy task. He underscored the so-called "free-rider" problem that creates a hurdle for interest groups pursuing collective benefits for their membership. Viewing individuals as "rational decision makers" and using a "rational economic man" model, Olson noted that people will not join organizations when they can enjoy whatever collective goals are obtained, such as those resulting from favorable legislation, which might be the case for registered nurses, without bearing the costs of participation in terms of time and money. This so-called "free-rider" problem is especially critical for large organizations such as the ANA. The larger the group, the less likely people are to think their contributions will have an impact on the group's success. Because of this attitude, people often refrain from seeking membership. Thus, group formation and survival are particularly delicate in nature.

Difficulties relating to group organization may also be highlighted from another perspective. C. S. Weissert and W. G. Weissert (1996) observe: " Some of the nation's strongest groups are weakened in their bargaining ability by their diverse membership. For groups representing a large, diverse membership, developing and maintaining a policy focus that satisfies all members can be tough . . ." (p. 136). The noted problem is a real one for associations embracing various types, even if they all belong to the same profession. A dominant theme pervading the interest group literature is that a major determinant of influence is the close relation between cohesion and the access that associations have to decision makers.

Of all the organizations in the interest group universe, according to Feldstein (1988), those related to nursing have encountered the most difficulty in organizing their members. This is attributed to the fact that the members' interests are ". . . not as similar nor as singular as in other professions" (pp. 54–55). Organization is a difficult task because there are more constituents to organize. Moreover, they are not completely aware of the benefits of membership and the incentives are few. He notes that nursing organizations have been reticent to act as unionizing agents. However, they have been forced to do so as other unions have entered their terrain. He sternly warns: ". . . Unless nurse associations can replicate the unions in overcoming the free rider problem, it is unlikely that the reasons for low membership in state and national nursing associations can be easily overcome" (p. 55).

One empirical study compared teachers, engineers, and nurses in terms of their relationship with their official professional organization. It was found that nurses demonstrate less of a propensity to join. The American Nurses Association is similar in terms of its constituency to the National Education Association. Both are hybrids between a professional organization and a labor union. The proportion of educators joining their professional group was much greater than that for nursing. Moreover, it was noted that those nurses who do join their official association are significantly less active in it than teachers and engineers are in theirs. Obviously, this situation has economic implications and consequences for the effectiveness of the groups (Cutting, 1982; Hanley, 1987). It is generally acknowledged that an entity is more likely to exercise power if its membership is large and well distributed.

ANA Structure

The structure of an organization affects the relationship it has with its members as well as their participation in its activities. In 1982 in an attempt to combine unity with diversity, the ANA adopted a federated and indirect structure. The organization became a union of component professional groups, which include the geographically based state nurses associations (SNAs), comprised of district nurses associations; multistate nurses associations, American nurses overseas associations, and a unit for active duty military nurses. Prior to 1982, an individual could join the ANA directly or could affiliate with the SNA or the district association without becoming a member of the national organization. After the structural adjustment, membership is achieved through affiliation with one of the constituent parts. Thus, there is not a direct link between the individual and the national community because members form a professional community with the aid of another social grouping—usually the SNA. Membership is termed indirect. The federated and indirect structure model assigned a new role to the SNAs. Having more independence and autonomy in the new organizational arrangements, they were to exert greater control and influence. Moreover, it was believed that they would be able to recruit more members. Obviously, this did not occur.

As part of its new look, the 1999 ANA House of Delegates approved the development of a federal constituency for active-duty military nurses, the Federal Nurses Association. This innovation, open only to nurses employed by the United States Army, Navy, Air Force and the Public Health Service, is part of a major effort to increase ANA membership. The potential pool for new members is considerable, numbering approximately 12,000 persons (American Nurses Association, 2001). Only about 1,500 military nurses had belonged to SNAs. This situation resulted primarily from the fact that ANA bylaws only provided for a geographically based constituent member, as previously discussed. Also, nurses on active duty experience frequent relocations due to the nature of their employment. This does not allow for an intense identification with a particular state. Hence, most military nurses did not seek SNA membership. However, so as not to ruffle the feathers of the SNAs, all members of the new federal constituency will be linked to an SNA. With the creation of the new unit, SNAs are now formally referred to as constituency member associations (CMAs).

This structural change has advantages for all concerned parties. For the ANA, it diversifies its membership, enhances opportunities to increase its rank and file and, in turn, its financial resources. There is also the possibility of greater collaboration with the Federal Nursing Chiefs who use ANA practice standards and guidelines and support the baccalaureate requirement for entry into practice (American Nurses Association, 2001; "ANA at Work," 1999). Military nurses as well have new opportunities. They have a forum to collectively address issues related to their unique work environment and patient population. Moreover, they have a voice and representation not previously available.

As Duverger (1954) observes in a political science classic, the indirect structure has implications for solidarity within the organization and for the notion of community. As in the case of a political party organized on an indirect basis, the nature of the political bond and true participation in the life of the community are negatively affected.

Links between the individual and the national community, in this case the ANA, are tenuous at best. This, in part, might account for the fact that the participation of members in the ANA is low. It might also, partially explain why in the aforementioned comparison of nurses with teachers and engineers, it was found that nurses were significantly less active in professional organizations.

ANA Councils

One mechanism in the ANA structure that afforded members an opportunity for participation was the council. More specifically, according to Article XII of the bylaws, this organizational unit allowed members to take part ". . . in the improvement or advancement of the profession in an area of nursing practice or interest" (American Nurses Association, 1991, pp. 23–24). The number of councils was determined by the ANA board of directors. Until 1992 there were eleven councils (Community Health Nurses, Computer Applications in Nursing, Continuing Education and Staff Development, Cultural Diversity in Nursing, Gerontological Nursing, Maternal–Child Nursing, Medical-Surgical Nursing Practice, Nurse Researchers, Nurses in Advanced Practice, Nursing Administration, Psychiatric and Mental Health Nursing), all of which were centrally organized at the national level. As is evident from their names, their focus was categorical reflecting the populations served, practice arenas or roles inside or outside of direct clinical practice. Some had a narrow scope overlapping with specialty practice groups, while others were broader in nature. Whereas one centered on the direct clinical practice role, others were outside of it. Moreover, a few were identified with areas that cut across the nursing discipline, such as cultural diversity in nursing and computer applications. Council memberships were considerably uneven, ranging from very small to quite large. Those with the smallest memberships were overconsuming scarce resources. The councils undertook administrative chores such as collecting dues, generating newsletters and so on, with little responsibility for securing valuable ways and means to make themselves self-sufficient. In short, they were a drain on the total structure and it was believed that these units did not operate in a way that was congruent with previous organizational changes (Shaver,

1994). It was decided to retain the councils, reduce them in number and to alter their function somewhat. They became six in number (Acute Care Nursing Practice, Advanced Nursing Practice, Community-Based Primary and Long-Term Care Practice, Nursing Research, Nursing Systems and Administration, Professional Nursing Education and Development) and SNA members could join two ("Purposes Outlined," 1994). Commenting on this modification, Shaver (1994) observes:

> Now the councils are resources . . . for advancing the health-care reform agenda, for coalescing information across SNAs on issues that cut across most or all states, to promulgate standards of direct or indirect clinical practice and certification and articulate positions of the association on behalf of the SNAs regarding public policy and resource allocation with national impact. (p. 11)

The survey sought to elicit information about participation in council activities. In an open-ended question, respondents were asked to specify the names of the councils to which they belong and to indicate their level of involvement according to a specific scale. Just above the space in which respondents were to supply this information, the survey instrument listed the councils with their new names. It is noteworthy that in responding to this question, respondents, for the most part, wrote in the names that these units had under the old arrangement. Such an occurrence could indicate that the ANA was not totally effective in communicating the new structure to its clientele. In terms of membership, by far the most popular units were Nursing Research; Community-Based, Primary and Long-Term Care Practice, and Professional Nursing Education and Development, in that order. On the other hand, Nursing Systems and Administration attracted no members from this sample. Twenty-two percent of the respondents claimed membership in the council structure and two percent of this group belonged to two councils. Seventy-eight percent had no affiliation with the council structure. In terms of level of involvement in a particular council, in all cases, a majority of the respondents indicated inactive status, meaning that they paid dues but rarely attended meetings, and so on. The sample definitely did not take advantage of the opportunity to participate.

The council structure was precarious. It became more tenuous as human and financial resources became more limited. In light of cutback management at the 1999 House of Delegates, the councils and other participatory organs were abolished. They were replaced with a single unit, the Congress on Nursing Practice and Economics. This body performs the same functions as the eliminated councils and is to create ad hoc issue groups as needed, thus justifying the label "adhocracy" model.

Specialty Organizations

The professionalization project implies a significant degree of specialization. As their knowledge base expands, occupations usually divide into a series of subgroups. This happened in the case of nursing. It has been reported that a student once remarked: "[I]t seems that every time nurses identify a problem, their first action is to form a new organization" (Ellis & Hartley, 1995, p. 449). There is some truth to this statement, even though it is exaggerated. This internal differentiation profoundly affects interprofessional relations and in its extreme can seriously weaken jurisdictional controls. Special-interest organizations are not new to the nursing profession. The earliest ones began in the second decade of this century with the formation of the Industrial Nurses' Club in 1915. However, it is since the middle of the last century that nursing specialty organizations have blossomed. They came into being either as a splinter group that separated from the ANA or as units that were born independently as the profession became more specialized. The birth and growth of these associations is natural in that they reflect the heterogeneity of the profession. Nurses do not have identical interests. As noted elsewhere in this work, they have always been split internally. Having a variety of practice settings and different levels of education, they divide on the basis of education or site of employment with variations in levels of control and autonomy. Having diverse educational backgrounds, not all nurses possess the same skills. For example, those with baccalaureate and master's degrees practice with a great deal of autonomy and in addition to providing bedside care in complicated circumstances, they are prepared to plan for the management and evaluation of patient care in cooperation with personnel in other disciplines. Nurse practitioners are specialists who possess advanced clinical knowledge in a particular area. Associate degree-prepared nurses practice with less autonomy and demonstrate diverse technical talents for bedside care.

Approximately two-thirds of the nursing population works in an acute-care setting, the hospital. Even those, however, may be divided on a generalist–specialist basis and again as to a specific specialty such as pediatric nursing, critical care nursing, and so forth. The rest of the population works in other sites, such as academia, long-term care facilities, public health agencies, educational institutions, physicians' offices, clinics, industry, and the home, to cite a few. Again, this constituency may be divided on a generalist–specialist basis. Having a galaxy of employment opportunities, it is natural that members of the profession, depending on their place of employment, make unique and varied contributions to the health care delivery system and its outputs, and develop special interests. With the passage of time it is also natural that people working in a particular area have a greater identification with it than with their profession in general. They become committed to it and often their primary concern is to advance its interest. Thus, specialty nursing associations were established to meet the specific needs of nurses working in a particular sector. In the words of one member, ". . . [S]pecialty organizations attract many nurses because they can appeal to that special sense of what you do" ("Membership Matters," 1995, p. 14). Representing more accurately their professional roles, nurses belonging to each of these associations manifest a greater similarity of interest than those under the umbrella of the ANA. Some of these organizations are completely independent, while others are affiliated with another association. In terms of membership, some restrict it to nurses, whereas others, in addition to nurses, admit technical-medical personnel.

These diverse groups internal to the profession assume the character of social movements. They develop distinctive identities, a sense of the past, and goals for the future. Their activities secure their institutional position and aid in the implementation of their objectives. Their behavior affects the organization of the profession as a whole. It moves relationships within a profession and also influences relations with external forces (Bucher & Strauss, 1961).

All of these special-interest groups perform certain common functions. In addition to furnishing a forum so that colleagues may exchange experiences and problems concerned with a specific specialty or interest, they are involved with continuing-education endeavors, standard setting, leadership development and, in some cases, certification of specialty practice. Many nurses are of the opinion that their benefits from this type of association are greater than those from the ANA. Not only might this be true, but also the cost has usually been less. Dues of the specialty groups have generally been lower than those of the ANA. In addition, these single-purpose organizations, for the most part, have quicker response mechanisms, in part, because they are centrally and directly organized and they focus on selected issues. Recognizing the complexity of the health care delivery system and its technology, and the need to excel in clinical practice in a specific area, if a choice must be made, many nurses prefer to identify with specialty organizations rather than the ANA. Thus, as the latter was experiencing a decline in membership, the former were realizing an increase (Hriceniak, 1994; Zerwekh & Claborn, 1994). In fact, these specialty groups have emerged as the primary identity of many nurses. The ANA is currently attempting to establish a mechanism to encourage increased CMA membership of nurses in the specialty organizations.

There is a galaxy of active nursing specialty associations. Few professions have so many different groups trying to represent it. All of these compete for members. As noted earlier, historically nurses' earnings have not been high. Thus, often the decision of whether to join a specialty association and how many to join has been an economic as well as a philosophical issue. However, it is noteworthy that an increase in salaries did not lead to a significant change in participation in professional nursing organizations (Ellis & Hartley, 1995). In this sample, 32% was affiliated with a specialty association. Of this group eight percent belonged to two, and under one percent to three. In comparing the respondents' membership in the ANA and specialty associations, the higher percentage in the case of the latter demonstrates their attractiveness. Membership was held in eighteen different specialty organizations, the most popular of which, as one might expect, given the focus of this study, was the American Association of Colleges of Nursing. Membership was concentrated in this organization. Other popular ones included the Association for Women's Health, Obstetric and Neonatal Nurses; Oncology Nursing Society, and the American Academy of Nurse

Practitioners. It has been noted that nurses display less of a propensity to join professional associations than other professionals. Comparative studies of nurses, engineers and teachers have demonstrated that nurses belong to significantly fewer organizations than members of the other two professions. Seventy percent of nurses were members of only one or two associations, whereas the percentage for teachers was 58 and that for engineers was 56. Over 40% of the engineers and teachers belonged to three or more organizations versus 30% of nurses (Hanley, 1987). Thus, not only are the percentages related to organizational affiliations in this study low in comparison to those for other professionals, but they are low in comparison to the rest of the nursing profession. In terms of this sample's level of involvement in specialty organizations, active membership status was somewhat higher (22%) in the specialty organizations than in the ANA, again indicating the lure of the specialty orientation. Also, a leadership role accounted for five percent and nine percent respectively of the members in local and/or state units and at the national level. If these figures are compared to those for other professions, it is evident that nurses in this sample are significantly less active in their professional associations than are teachers and engineers.

In addition to organizations that focus on a particular clinical or functional specialty, special-interest nursing associations also include those that are based on meritorious performance, and ethnic, racial and religious identities. The survey instrument elicited information concerning identification with this type of special-interest group. Respondents exhibited a preference for an affiliation with this category as opposed to that with a specialty orientation. Seventy-two percent held membership in one of these groups and 10% identified with two. As in the case of the specialty associations, less than one percent of the sample held membership in three groups. The association that attracted by far the most members was Sigma Theta Tau International, the international honor society of nursing. Membership in other organizations in this category was minuscule in comparison to that of the honor society. In terms of level of involvement, as in other instances, most responses centered on an inactive status.

Nurses have a galaxy of organizations competing for their membership dollars and participation. Questions have been raised concerning the rapport between these entities and the overlapping of function. It is generally recognized that membership in these various professional bodies impinges negatively on professional unity. Perhaps the only thing that is more destructive than this is the number of professionals without any professional identity reflected in a collegial body (Perrucci, 1973). This was the case for 15% of the respondents to the survey. Although each subgroup tends to focus on its own interests, members in the broader profession are of the opinion that they do not lose very much by this lack of cohesion. This is a critical matter. It is true that these various associations have enhanced the group consciousness of nurses and have provided a structure through which it can express itself. However, at the same time they have been divisive. Not only do they vie with each other for members, they also compete for a role as the leader of the profession as a whole. The question becomes whether these organizations will look beyond their own specific goals and unify around issues of importance to all nurses. Moreover, the claim to trust and autonomy, the basis of professionalism, is undermined. In the future, with more complexity in the health care delivery system and technological change, it is likely that these groups will continue to increase in number.

The relationship between the various nursing groups is permeated with competition rather than cooperation. The contest focuses on membership and other scarce resources as well as policy issues. Naturally, this has damaged the influence of nursing in the political arena. Organizational duplication, divisiveness and turf squabbles have hindered nursing interest groups' political capabilities. One nurse has observed:

> As nurses, we sometimes shoot ourselves in the foot. We look at the things that make us different—not what makes us the same. We need to focus on the reasons we all went into nursing—to care for our patients, to help and assist people, to make the quality of their life better, to move them along the health continuum. We need to find that common ground where we can agree on things. ("Membership Matters," 1995, p. 14)

In part, some of these difficulties were caused by the lack of formal channels for cooperative efforts. In an attempt to rectify this situation of organizational disarray and tension between diverse nursing agendas, alliances among nursing organizations have been forged. Examples include the National Federation of Specialty Nursing Organizations, Nursing Organization Liaison Forum, and the Tri-Council for Nursing, all coalitions of nursing associations, as is evident from their names, and all relatively young organizations in terms of age. Each of these will be briefly discussed in turn.

Although it was active under another name in the 1970s, the National Federation of Specialty Nursing Organizations (NFSNO), a loosely structured alliance of clinical specialty associations commonly referred to as the Federation, was formally born in 1981 with the scope of achieving a unified voice for specialty nursing. Its membership consists of groups diverse in size that must meet certain criteria. Presently the organization consists of 32 groups classified as regular members and three who are affiliate members, the latter fulfilling most, but not all, of the membership requirements. In addition to advancing specialty practice through educational efforts and providing a reference point for those interested in specific nursing specialties, it serves as a mechanism for networking, dealing with issues of common concern among nursing specialty organizations and building collaborative efforts. Also of importance to it is information exchange with appropriate groups on cogent issues and influencing policy-making on matters related to specialty nursing.

Another mechanism for nurturing collaboration among national nursing associations is the National Organization Liaison Forum (NOLF). It was created as an organizational unit within the ANA to furnish a forum for discussion between nursing associations and the ANA. More specifically, its purpose is to promote, under the aegis of the ANA, discussion of issues of interest to all sectors of the nursing profession as well as concerted action on issues of professional policy and national health policy of mutual concern. Thus, its focus and membership base are broader than those of the Federation. NOLF has counted as its members national nursing organizations, the ANA councils; the American Academy of Nursing, an entity for the recognition of professional merit; and special-interest nursing groups. There is an obvious duplication of effort in that it includes many organizations that are also part of the NFSNO alliance.

Originally the Tri-Council for Nursing, which was established in 1981, consisted of the ANA, the National League for Nursing, and the American Association of Colleges of Nursing. Within four years, the American Organization of Nurse Executives joined its ranks, but there was no title change in spite of the fact that with the additional member the unit was no longer a tri-council. In reality, the organization is an informal alliance among the presidents, presidents-elect and chief executive officers of the affiliated units. The structure was created because of the importance of establishing a unified approach to the critical nursing issues of the day and the need to respond in coherent fashion to multiple interdependencies. A specific objective of the organization is the facilitation of coordination and communication related to significant professional matters and endeavors as well as aiding with the conclusion of agreements on federal legislation of common concern. The agenda of the Tri-Council is distinguished from that of its counterparts in that it is less narrow in its focus. The issues that it confronts are more generic in nature.

Such alliances are important. Mechanisms that bring together a number of group leaders and identify common interests enhance the probability of a congruence between the policies they desire and the underlying attitudes of the proximate decision makers to whom they must appeal (Lindblom, 1968). Although these nursing coalitions have played an important role in the policy-making process, it is generally agreed that they possess much potential that has not been realized. Consistency in the collaborative approach is lacking and it is often not clear in specific instances if the associations individually and collectively represent a united front. As alliances, they frequently display independent interests and the need for defined policy priorities is evident. This makes it difficult to determine who is the actual spokesperson for the nursing profession. It has also been suggested that there should be more unity and commitment of human resources within and among the alliances (Hall-Long, 1995a; Kuhn, 1986). A joint task force is presently examining various ways for the ANA and the specialty organizations to structure relationships so that all sectors of the profession will be united and the strengths of each one will be accentuated. This is not an easy task.

The fact that these structures were created demonstrates that the nursing leaders understand the need to unify around issues of mutual concern. Given the dates of the births of these coalitions, this requirement was recognized in different sectors of the profession at the same time. Failure to realize this need would have been perilous. Two members of the profession have correctly observed, "If our nursing organizations continue to fight among themselves and appear to be waging self-serving battles within the health care arena, others will simply take over . . ." (Hillestad & Hawken, 1996, p. 128). The value of these alliances is considerable, even though they have not completely solved the problem for which they were created. In a speech to the 2000 House of Delegates meeting, Linda J. Stierle, ANA Executive Director and Chief Executive Officer warned, ". . . [I]t is past the time when we can afford to continue to focus on our differences and let them drive us apart and weaken and dilute the strength of our voice" (*ANA 2000*, 2000).

PROFESSIONAL NURSING ORGANIZATIONS: POTENTIAL AND REALITY

Such is the sketch map of the territory occupied by professional nursing organizations, drawing attention to the principal ones and their dimensions. In spite of the variety of these organizations and their overtures to potential members, it is quite clear that this sample, in terms of its behavior, does not perceive the benefits of membership. These associations may be compared to a kaleidoscope in that they are of many shapes and forms, dynamic and constantly changing as a result of stimuli from inside and outside the profession. Serving as a mirror for the profession, they have reflected its growing complexity, increasing in number and becoming more specialized in scope. An attempt has been made to overcome the resulting centrifugal forces of this arrangement with the establishment of organizational vehicles for consensus.

A danger signal is that groups continue to form and many in the universe contend that they will remain autonomous units. On the other hand, one observer notes that nursing organizations are developing a trust in the group process and a readiness to reconsider a meaningful partnership between the ANA and the specialty organizations (P. M. Kelly, 1999). A critical question to resolve is: Do these groups speak for nursing in addition to the ANA or in place of the ANA? Other questions to be answered include: Does the ANA's major role lie in the area of policy formation and lobbying in the interests of all sectors of the profession at the national and subnational units of government? Is the principal function of the specialty organizations advancement of the body of knowledge of a specific specialty and the identification of issues that require the policy development efforts of the ANA? If these disparate groups do not agree on roles and continue to go their own way, ignoring global professional issues, and membership in the ANA continues to diminish, the sense that the profession is unable to confront other constituencies with one voice will undoubtedly increase.

Public displays of divisiveness within organized nursing reap significant political costs. Obviously, they compromise the effectiveness of the profession's interest articulation. Archer (1982) aptly notes: "Failure of a group, such as nursing, to unite its many internal factions . . . into a solid front, sets the group up for outside forces to use divide-and-conquer tactics on the group. Indeed, this is what is happening in nursing now" (p. 94). Although written several years ago, this observation is still cogent. Moreover, the economic incentive is important to the daily existence of professions. Wilsford (1991) writes: ". . . the more dominant the economic incentive, the easier the group may organize and maintain its membership. And the strategic position of the group may depend most on the economic function the group performs in the society and economy" (p. 89). The nursing profession has not been income producing and, thus, the economic incentive is not as great as in other professions. It has not stemmed the tide of proliferation.

Obviously, some health associations, such as the American Medical Association (AMA), have been more successful in the legislative realm than others such as the ANA. Feldstein (1988) attributes supremacy to the relative income of the membership. Arguing from an economic perspective, as does Wilsford (1991), that the income of the rank and file is the most useful predictor for judging success of an interest group in the legislative marketplace, he notes that in the post–World War II era physicians have earned excess rates of return. These were higher than what it would have cost to produce the same number of doctors. In the case of the nurses, the rate of return is lower than that gained in other professions with comparable training. Nurses have failed to earn excess rates of return, which, it is argued, has hindered their influence on policy and role in the policy arena. In the real world economic advantage goes hand in hand with respectability. The traditional strength of the AMA has been attributed to its undeniable authority and influence over the medical profession, its economic position and the social prestige of the physician. Moreover, its membership base afforded organized medicine greater potential influence than that of other professional organizations.

For successful interest articulation, an interest sector must be mobilized. To achieve this status a constituency should possess a centralized structure and a high rate of membership. Additional requirements, among others, include the capacity to represent the membership with the government and to speak authoritatively on its behalf. Having this last ability means that the interest sector involved can guarantee the cooperation of its members in the implementation of any agreements it concludes. It is quite evident that these requisites do not apply to organized nursing. As noted elsewhere in this work, it is at odds with itself. It is plagued by fragmentation, divisiveness over issues, and internal conflicts that are reflected in the galaxy of competing professional organizations with very low membership levels.

Other occupations, such as law and medicine, have traditionally been characterized by a significant degree of homogeneity and consensus. According to Goode (1969), they form "communities within the community." Among the membership there is a consensus of identity, values, definition of role and interests. However, at the same time there is room for diversity, even to the point of conflict. The key element is that there is a steadfast core that denotes the profession and departures from it are not permanent (Atkinson, 1993). In its recent history the AMA has weathered several storms. Although it has emerged battered, it has survived. In fact, of all the health care associations, it has been considered the most successful in terms of dealing with a heterogeneous membership. This success has been attributed to its ability to attend to the common economic interests of all physicians (Feldstein, 1988). In the case of organized nursing with its many deviations, the question becomes, can the ANA, as it is, survive as the official national professional organization of nursing in this age of specialization? It has encountered trouble in defending the interests of the entire nursing profession. It is difficult for a professional association to be all things to all sectors of the profession. To be a viable organization, will the ANA have to follow in the AMA's footsteps and rely on a common set of economic interests in the framework of an increasingly diverse and dwindling membership?

Respondents to the survey did not give the ANA and one of its components (the New York SNA) a very good report card. One's overall evaluation of an interest group will depend on the person's perception of the leaders' influence on policy and the evaluator's relationship with the group's leadership. Respondents were asked to rate nursing's current influence in policy development at the state and national levels of government. The rank order in both cases was fair, poor and good. In terms of percentages these preferences translate respectively to 49%, 29%, and 22% at the state level and to 54%, 28% and 19% at the national level. These evaluations can be used, in part, to explain low membership levels. Obviously, people will not join an organization that they perceive as having stubbed its toe. In both cases an overwhelming majority of the sample (78% at the state level and 82% at the national level) rated interest articulation on behalf of nursing by the officially recognized association as less than good.

These orientations contrast with those manifested by members of the ANA's "Speak Up" market research panels consisting of various nurse market segments such as executives, educators, staff nurses, advanced practitioners, self-employed nurses and recent graduates. In a survey, the group wholeheartedly endorsed the efforts of the ANA. Eighty-eight percent was positive about its political impact ("Speak Up," 1994). In a more recent poll of SNA members, 81%, as opposed to 67% three years earlier, gave the association high grades for its performance and especially for its political endeavors, which included lobbying Congress and shaping legislation affecting nurses and patients ("SNA Members," 1999). These stances again indicate the strong relationship between membership in an organization and one's evaluation of it.

Data obtained from this survey indicate that there are obstacles to the advancement of the nursing profession as far as interest articulation is concerned. In the first place, there is uncertainty about an active role for the sample as well as the entire profession via participation in professional associations. Moreover, many of the interest-group resources that are important for impacting on various phases of the decision-making process, such as the constituency's ability to mobilize members, numbers, the internal cohesion of the group as well as coalitions, have not been solidified. Professional nursing's potential has been diluted, given the nature of its interest-group arena.

THE INTEREST GROUP UNIVERSE

It must be recognized that these professional nursing organizations do not operate in a vacuum. They must be seen in relation to the policy community in general, and the prevailing interest group environment and that of the health care sector, in particular. Advanced industrial societies have experienced a systematic value change (Flanagan, 1982; Inglehart, 1990), which has been reflected in the institutions of the political process and in a new alignment of preferences or interests. In recent years there have been significant changes in the power and influence of interest groups in the political system and especially in the health care sector. Interest groups have always been important in American politics. However, as the scope of government has expanded, so has their role and number. There has been a dramatic increase in interest advocacy in various policy domains and a concomitant augmentation in the number of interest groups. This advocacy explosion resulted from a variety of factors, including among other things, in addition to the extension of government activities and their proliferation, group reactions to particular events and to each other, the growth of adversary organizations, changes in the law facilitating group formation, the advancement of technology, and mutations in the social and political environment. Although many of the current associations were born after World War II, for the most part, this group explosion took place between 1960 and 1980 (Schlozman & Tierney, 1986; Walker, 1983).

One of its unique features is the significance of citizen groups that are prominent actors in the policy-making process at all levels of government and in administrative boards (Ingram & Smith, 1993). Many of these groups were spawned by a general social reform movement inspired ". . . by advocates of numerous broad interests common to all citizens or very large groups of them" (Lucco, 1992, p. 242). These broad interests, which include those of consumers or environmentalists, for example, are labeled public interests. It was argued that these widely held interests were neglected by the political establishment. Frequently groups reflecting them are motivated by a single issue, a cause or ideological concern and, as opposed to other associations, they do not have an occupational basis for membership. People join interest groups to achieve different types of rewards. There are (1) material or tangible rewards that can often be translated into monetary terms, (2) selective rewards available only to members of the group, (3) solidary or social rewards deriving from an association with group activities, and (4) purposive or expressive rewards affiliated with ideological or issue-oriented objectives that offer no significant tangible benefits to members. Rather than identifying with the material and selective benefits of the traditional groups, the public interests affiliate with solidary and purposive returns. They are able to maintain themselves because of the combined efforts of people who are disposed to work long and hard in the interests of a cause. This dedication results in self-gratification from joint endeavors to accomplish a strongly believed-in end. In the associations based on material and selective benefits, political factors are more directly connected to the size, structure and operation of the entity. On the other hand, the units that seek a collective good, the achievement of which will not selectively and materially benefit the membership, are able to establish a more dynamic organization in which politics, political preferences and group goals are more centrally determining factors (Moe, 1980; Olson, 1965; Sabatier, 1992).

A galaxy of public interests took its place alongside the more traditional formations, changing the basic nature of the interest group universe as well as the political agenda, which, in addition to the traditional economic and security issues, includes new concerns. Conflict now involves a different set of issues, such as environmental ones, those related to minority rights, and social equality, among others. All of these sectors relate to health. The political realm features a new dimension labeled the New Politics (Dalton, 1996). In the modern interest group arena these noted recent changes have opened up the political process by broadening the base of interest-group participation. In a sense, politics has become more representative than ever before. In this framework not only did the nature of the groups, their number, and issues of concern change, but there is heightened competition among them.

Many of these tendencies are reflected in the health care arena. The extent of the interest group explosion varied from one policy domain to another and it was particularly acute in the health care sector. The number of associations went from 674 in 1960 to 3,971 in 1992, representing a change of 589.3%. This compares with a growth rate of 169.4% in trade associations, 318.7% of groups in agriculture, and 565.7% in educational and cultural organizations (Baumgartner & Talbert, 1995). Growth in the health care domain clearly outdistanced all others. Moreover, health care units have become idiosyncratic and fragmented. They are no longer the monoliths they once were. Like nursing, many, such as organized medicine, and the drug, insurance, and hospital industries, have experienced divisions in their ranks, reflecting significant shifts in market conditions, government policies and public attitudes. In the new health care interest-group universe, the larger umbrella or peak associations, like the ANA or the AMA, exist side by side with others having a narrower focus. The former no longer dominate the entire agenda of health issues. Their orientations tend to be more general in nature, whereas those of the other organizations are more focused or specific. Obviously, the positions adopted reflect the membership base. In addition, some of these new associations are public-interest organizations. There is no health group that claims to speak for the entire health policy community. The new groups took their place in the health policy domain at the expense of the traditional ones, making it one of highly visible groups with many participants. In the health sector there has been strength in terms of numbers. It has been remarked that "there is no issue of public policy in which the sheer strength of those special interests have so overwhelmed the process as in . . . health care. . . ." (Seelye, 1994, p. A1).

This larger range of permanently organized interests, characterized by diversity and conflict, has impacted the policy-making process. It has tempered congressional control over policy outcomes. Given the nature of group conflict, more policy decisions take place on the floor of the Congress than in congressional committees. This ". . . does not allow for coherence, attention to detail, or controls by substantive experts . . ." (R.A. Smith, 1995, p. 114). Thus, many critical choices are left to the executive branch of government. Another change in the health care interest group universe concerns finances. An increase in the number of health care associations has meant more money is available for purposes of influencing the decision-making process. Such spending continues to escalate. Health care interest groups are among the most well-endowed.

Representational communities consist of all the organized interests in a specific policy domain. These interests may be divided into two categories: the stakeholders—those who tend to favor the status quo because of the benefits they reap from it—and the stake challengers—those who desire change because the existing situation is not beneficial to them. Relationships between these forces within the health care representational community have not remained static. Three distinct stages in the community's development may be identified. Up through the 1950s the stakeholders were allied and in command. For all practical purposes, the stake challengers were nonexistent. Thus, the community was homogeneous and labeled a block with the AMA solidly entrenched at the helm. No other voluntary association commanded such power or enjoyed more freedom from formal control. Through the medical press, group sanctions, expulsion, boycott, and other disciplinary techniques, the leaders of organized medicine were able to mold the opinions of American physicians. Capitalizing on its latent strength, the AMA skillfully applied the resources at its disposal to fashion health care policy according to its wishes. Its command traditionally relied on a combination of the pen, the sword and old-fashioned politics ("The American Medical Association," 1954; Garceau, 1940).

At the dawn of the 1960s and throughout the 1970s changes took place in the health care interest-group universe. Health care politics became more and more polarized as well-organized stake challengers faced the allied stakeholders. The representational community consisted of a dyad of two opposing coalitions. At this time the domain was more conflict ridden than it is today. In the next decade and into the 1990s the nature of health care interest-group politics changed dramatically. Many of the existing political alliances were transformed as a result of the development of managed care and changes in the economics of health care, cost shifting, and insurance arrangements. Tensions within the ranks of the stakeholders obliterated their cohesiveness and created competition among the various components. Meanwhile, the stake challengers increased in number and became more resilient, vocal and vigorous. Various groups issued divergent calls for change in the health care arena and of special significance was a severe decline in the ability of organized medicine to obstruct policy initiatives. Moreover, the latter's principal representative, the AMA, no longer enjoys dominance in medical decision making or a political monopoly in the world of the providers. Its vision of physician unity has been shattered. The influence of medical interest groups is no longer uniform. On some issues their demands are taken seriously and on others they are rejected. This, in part, resulted from the steady increase in health care costs and the resulting emphasis on cost containment as a policy objective. A spotlight was focused on the incomes of the health professions in general and, in particular, those of physicians. Moreover, there were transformations in consumer expectations, attitudes and behavior, the emergence of a new equilibrium within the medical profession, and challenges from other health care professions. Overall the representational network became loosely structured and, containing various types of groups with distinctly different views, heterogeneous. There being no health group that transcends the policy domain and claims to speak for the entire policy community, the level of acrimony that characterizes health politics is lower than it might be, if such a peak association existed (Baumgartner & Talbert, 1995; Jacobs, 1993; Mueller, 1993; Peterson, 1993; Salisbury, Heinz, Laumann, & Nelson, 1987; Tousijn, 2000).

INTEREST GROUPS AND THE POLICY PROCESS

Interest groups must also be seen in terms of their relationship with the political system they must penetrate to realize their objectives. Given that all do not enjoy equal access, it is imperative to maneuver and to fashion continuous relationships with policy makers to gain access more easily. An ideal arrangement for an interest group is a subgovernment or iron triangle. This three-way arrangement connects interests external to the government, in this case the stakeholders; an executive branch agency; and congressional committees or subcommittees in ways that routinize policy making and benefit those involved. All three constituents work by consensus to make policy in a particular area. Thus, a small group of actors dominate policy development. These impregnable iron triangles have controlled many policy domains, including health care. It was through this type of arrangement that the AMA and its allies were able to master the policy-making process. Such a mechanism, in part, explains the lack of radical change in a policy sector. In this fixed combination of public power and private interests that does not change over time, all participants benefit from the status quo and, therefore, resist changes in policies. It is clear that the principle of political equality is violated in this policy-making model. A privileged few enjoy access to the system and there is a frequent exclusion of majorities such as nurses.

As a result of the noted changes in the interest-group universe, some policy areas became populated by so many diverse participants adhering to contrasting views that they could not be managed by an iron triangle. Thus, subgovernment politics evolved into issue or network politics in some sectors. This was the case in the health care arena. "An issue network is a shared-knowledge group that ties together large numbers of participants with common technical expertise" (Berry, 1989, p. 174). Issue networks consist of the same actors that are on the iron triangle stage, interest groups, bureaucrats and legislators, but they are more extensive and diverse. Any actors who participate in the development of particular policies are included. Whereas subgovernments are simple and defined with clarity, issue networks are not. Participants come and go depending on the issue involved. This formation is more accessible to new participants than the iron triangle. The scope and confines of the community are determined by a shared focus of the members on certain policy issues, but with diverse perspectives, shared information and expertise, and competing stakes in the policy outcome (Peterson, 1993). Its structure is looser, more nebulous, less predictable and more fluid than that of its predecessor. Networks change as new groups gain prominence depending on the issue being discussed. Each group's role and degree of influence are modified as new policies are debated.

Although some groups, such as the AMA, hospital groups, the major insurance companies, members of congressional committees, and the Department of Health and Human Services, are regular participants in most issue networks, they are not dominant as they were in the iron-triangle model. The health policy domain has become increasingly complex. It involves a wide array of issues and participants. An opponent in one instance might be an ally in another. Different networks consisting of diverse actors constantly emerge. The wide variety of actors involved and the fluid relationships between them enhance the opportunity for change in policy. In the health care arena the antireform alliance is no longer an autonomous actor in the policy-making process. The number and types of active participants in health policy making have expanded well beyond the once-dominant provider interest groups. Given the nature of issue networks and the incrementalism of American public policy, meaning that change should take place in incremental stages without changing the fundamental design of the structure of the policy domain, it is likely that various initiatives will focus on specific aspects of health care delivery rather than the total system. Any discussion of health care reform will be ". . . dominated by a kaleidoscope of variously focused coalitions, each composed of subsets of interest groups" (Kosterlitz, 1994, p. 412). The emergence of the issue network and its intragovernmental and extragovernmental expansion have provided a refreshing and exciting inertia and new resources for policy development in the health care arena.

In part, because of developments within the interest-group universe, the possibilities for reform in health care are greater. The traditional barriers to changes in health policy have been tempered with the evolution of issue networks and a combination of long-term social, economic, and political alterations. In the past, health care did not enjoy a high priority on the public agenda. Such is no longer the case. Many nonprovider groups, such as the American Association of Retired Persons, have continually highlighted the subject. The public's attitude on the matter has changed. Its attention has focused on various facets of health policy. Even though President Clinton's efforts at health care reform were not successful, health care is still a pressing issue.

Although there are various models of policy making, the two basic perspectives presented here are often singled out for special attention. The power relationships affiliated with each one, plus the ranking of health care issues on the nation's political agenda, impact the role and activities of the various nursing organizations. In either case their task is formidable. Given the role of organized medicine and its allies in the iron triangle, principally the insurance industry and business, the exclusion of nursing organizations loomed large. On the other hand, on the stage of the issue networks, they are merely one of many characters in search of an author. Competition is keen. The specific behavior of respondents to the survey, as will be seen in subsequent chapters, and their lack of group orientation as evidenced in this chapter, have implications for interest-group politics and significant consequences for the success of nursing in the policy-making arena.

Chapter 3

Nurse Educators: Political Behavior and Public Policies

INTRODUCTION

Rapid and tumultuous changes in the health care industry result from policy choices at all levels of government. Nurses, regardless of their site of practice, are affected on a daily basis by politics. It impacts many issues of importance to them, such as the scope and site of practice, reimbursement, malpractice, licensure, education, and research, to cite a few. Moreover, the range of health-related subjects with which government is concerned has enlarged. Thus, the profession is increasingly fashioned by political decisions that are relevant to areas with which it is identified: the workplace, government, professional organizations, and the community at large. In this context nurses' political participation is vital to the attainment of professional and personal goals. Given the extent to which political decisions affect the profession, nursing is inseparable from politics that directly relates to professional status.

The public and, more specifically, nurse educators, have a plethora of opportunities as individuals or as group members to influence political decisions. Three models symbolize political linkages and the interaction between the public and its decision makers. In the first one, constituents, as individuals, using rewards and sanctions in the form of votes and campaign assistance among other activities, influence their representatives, who logically should take the constituents' preferences into account because of the damage or aid that they can deliver. The same methods may be used in connection with membership in or support for mediating groups such as interest associations or political parties that bring together people with common interests and preferences to be transmitted to political leaders. Again, it is assumed the elite will listen to these messages because of the possibility of sanctions. These models relate to direct influence in that pressure is directly exerted on representatives or candidates for public office. Constituent influence may also be of the indirect variety. This results when representatives act in accordance with constituent preferences either because they are of the same conviction or they believe that such preferences should prevail over their own. All of these models are interdependent. For example, the importance of the electoral linkage is related to group linkages that, in turn, are connected to the representative ones (Ippolito, Walker, & Kolson, 1976).

It is through role modeling that nurse educators can demonstrate the significance of political involvement to the profession and its future members. Moreover, as noted above, faculty role modeling of the knowledge, attitudes and behaviors associated with successfully impacting the political system is critical to the development of political competence. Most participants in the survey (79%) acknowledged faculty role modeling as the most effective strategy for involving students in policy development. Given their influence on future members of the profession, it is timely to examine the political involvement of nurse educators. This chapter has as its principal thrust the sample's political participation, political legislative knowledge base, and attitudes toward policy development.

POLITICAL PARTICIPATION

Consisting of many forms, political participation refers to individual activities in the political arena by citizens. A section of the survey was designed to elicit information concerning the respondents' identification with various participation modes. The most basic form of political participation is one central to theories of democratic control through elections: voting, an act that relates the individual to the political system, legitimizes the democratic process, and serves as a visible and symbolic component of political participation and strength. The ballot is an effective instrument of citizen participation. Assuming competition among the political parties contesting the election, voters have an opportunity to influence policy making in general and on a specific basis—issue by issue.

Elections are an important form of control. The amount of control they exercise depends on the type of policy involved. Sometimes the public is not interested in issues or it is not adequately informed. Thus, it exerts no immediate control. This is particularly true when the issues are very complex and technically sophisticated or they do not directly impinge on the individual voter. The public's judgment is usually retrospective on those issues that are debated and discussed during political campaigns. Consequently, leaders at first exercise considerable discretion in problem solving. Their performance and decision-making skills are reviewed and evaluated come election time. Rather than prescribing or proscribing specific policy initiatives, electors have an interest in the performance of the political parties or public officials in power. They issue rewards or sanctions through the ballot box. However, there are instances in which the public has exerted direct and immediate control over leadership initiatives (Ippolito et al., 1976; Smith, 1998). The act of voting is important because frequently it is the only political activity in which citizens engage.

A contemporary phenomenon is the politicization of women. They have become more important worldwide in the electoral arena. This assigns a new significance to the political activities of nurses, given the fact that theirs is a female profession. With over 2.2 million registered nurses in the United States working in health care, one out of every 100 adults is a nurse and one in 38 female voters is a nurse. Clearly, this is a political resource with great potential. Electoral activities are a vital strategy for interest groups. The importance of the ballot to the profession was recognized long ago by nursing leaders. Even before female suffrage received official professional support, one nurse leader vehemently argued: "Until we possess the ballot we shall not know when we may get up in the morning to find that all we had gained has been taken from us" (Lewenson, 1993, p. 227).

The United States is atypical in that voter turnout tends to be less than that in other countries. In many other nations turnout rates of

80% or more have been common. On the other hand, in the United States one hears the phrase "the vanishing electorate" or the "puzzle of participation" because voting is the only political activity for which there is evidence of a decline in participation in recent years. Changing demographic trends of voter turnout have fueled great debate. In the 1992 presidential election in which President Clinton was victorious, election turnout was at its highest in two decades—55%—and in the 1996 poll in which he was reelected, turnout registered 49%, the lowest since 1924. The turnout rate in the 1998 election cycle dropped to a low of 36% and in 2000, being a presidential election, it rose to about 51%. Electoral turnout is always greater in presidential contests. (Edwards, Wattenberg, & Lineberry, 2000; Greenberg & Page, 1993; "United States," 1996, 2000).

Anemic turnout rates result, in part, from the unique American system of voter registration in which the citizen must assume the initiative to register before an election. On the other hand, most often and specifically in nations with higher turnout rates, voter registration is the government's responsibility. The citizen only has to appear at the polls. In addition, in the United States strict requirements related to residency create barriers to participation. Moreover, Americans are saturated with elections. Having more voting opportunities than citizens of many other nations, often they tend to forfeit the advantages of electoral participation. Also, the choices offered electors in the United States are not as clear-cut as in other countries. Extreme parties on the left and right of the political continuum are minor parties and they do not threaten political stability. Consequently, the electoral stakes are less significant than elsewhere. This fact also impacts on the low turnout rate.

The nursing profession has a high percentage of practitioners who vote. As found in other studies (Creason, 1978), in this one, nurses voted in higher proportion than the population at large. Eighty-three percent of the respondents reported that they always go to the polls and 12% usually do so. The rest claimed they never vote (2%) or only vote occasionally (4%). Not all persons in these last two groups should be labeled apathetic. Some people do not go to the polls because they are satisfied with the government's performance. They only vote when they become dissatisfied. Others are completely alienated from the political system and, therefore, fail to vote. Overall, the political activism of the sample in regard to elections is evident. For it, voting is by far the most popular participation mode. It is an important method of citizen influence on policy. These results may be compared to a recent ANA poll of SNA members in which 76% of the sample voted in all elections (deVries, 1996). Income and occupation along with education are key predictors of levels of political participation. The critical factor in explaining voter turnout is level of formal education. Respondents in this study are more highly educated than the general population of registered nurses. Thus, one would expect their turnout rate to be greater.

Beyond voting there are other avenues of citizen participation in the play of power in policy making. Voter turnout is only one avenue through which citizens participate in electoral politics. Although most citizens have little impact on policy, extremely energetic folks with some competence, using strategies other than voting, can leave their mark. An extension of electoral participation that requires more initiative than voting is involvement in campaign activities. These include distribution of literature, organization of events, registration drives, telephone campaigns, and door-to-door canvassing, among other things. Predictors of this type of involvement are education and party attachment. The political skills and resources represented by education have more influence on participation rates. An individual exerts more political influence by becoming involved in a campaign than by voting. Moreover, campaign involvement conveys more information than voting (Dalton, 1996). Despite the low voter turnout levels in the United States, Americans are more likely than people in other nations to participate in election campaigns. In fact, they become involved at relatively higher levels. Whereas the number of citizens voting in presidential and midterm elections has decreased since the 1960s, participation in other dimensions of electoral politics has increased (Edwards et al., 2000; Shields & Goidel, 2000). Although men are more active in campaign activity than women, given their rate of voting, educational achievements, and party attachment, it could be anticipated that respondents to this survey would have gone beyond voting and taken an active role in interest articulation and these activities. Leavitt & Mason (1994) note that because of their "people skills," nurses are ideal campaign volunteers. They are capable communicators, able to juggle many tasks and deal with stress. However, this was not the case. Respondents to the survey were not activists.

Of the wide range of campaign activities, the one most engaged in by the sample was discussion of candidates without participation in formally organized efforts. As far as this activity is concerned, nurse educators are more active than the public at large. Only about a third of it engage in discussions of how to vote (Hrebenar, Burbank, & Benedict, 1999). On the other hand, 29% and 41% respectively of the sample reported they always or usually engage in dialogue related to candidates. Twenty-four percent claimed to occasionally do so and six percent never became involved. As for the last two groups, and especially the last one, it is noteworthy that one current of opinion believes that professionals are expected to keep their professional and partisan lives separate, maintaining silence on their political and personal views. Political action is deemed unprofessional, unwomanly and unnecessary. It does seem appropriate and opportune for professionals to articulate their opinions on candidates' orientations toward policy matters related to their profession, the societal need for which it was created, and the public good. They should enhance the public's cognizance of the issues in question. Historically nursing has failed to impart to the citizenry knowledge and opinions relevant to health. Moreover, it has been reported that many nurse educators are passive in discussions and in decision making. This is of limited or no political value (Deloughery & Gebbie, 1975; Lowery-Palmer, 1982). The public's awareness and understanding of the profession have been lessened. Nurses are in a strategic position to educate the citizenry and elected officials on health care issues because they are at the point of patient care. To one nurse leader this failure to engage in dialogue is baffling. She writes:

> There is an old Negro spiritual that says, "I couldn't keep it to myself." What keeps our words and our songs of the power of this profession tied up within the prison of our minds? For nursing professionalism to exist and thrive, we must engage our associations, colleagues, friends and enemies, relatives and communities in a continuing national dialogue about nursing and how we make a difference. (Malone, 1998, p. 5)

Nurses have an obligation to educate the public about their role. Public education is important to their autonomy and credibility. The public must be informed and must appreciate that nursing issues are their issues because resolution of these matters determines what type of care will be delivered and to whom. The message must be widely broadcast. By disseminating information to citizens, policy makers, business and insurance companies as well as other constituencies, nurses can have an impact on decision making. Relying on their education and experiences, they are well qualified to speak to services needed for specific populations, among other things. Moreover, the value of nursing's input is based on its societal mandate as the primary provider and coordinator of direct care and its patient advocate role. Seventy-six percent of the sample approved of activism in policy making for nurses. Furthermore, the generation of discussion on candidates and issues, in this case nursing and health care issues, is important to the vibrancy of democratic society. People having limited familiarity with broad issues often disenfranchise themselves, whereas extensive familiarity with issues is accompanied by high rates of participation (Lindblom, 1968).

Closely related to dialogue is public opinion, ". . . the complex of preferences expressed by a significant number of persons on an issue of general importance" (Hennessy, 1981, p. 8). Public policies represent governmental responses to human needs and desires. All public policies at one time were simply a private idea that came to be accepted by a large number of people. These private ideas, when aggregated, become proposals and when adopted by governmental authorities, public policies. Policy is sensitive to information, discussion, study and preferences, all of which are a part of public opinion whose real importance lies in the long road of transformation into public policy. The policy-making process is ". . . a representation of the way opinions are funded, interpreted, and given meaning as policies are arrived at through legislation, executive action and judicial action . . ." (Hennessy, p. 293). Political parties and interest groups represent stable linkages through which public opinion may be transmitted to government. Many interest groups incorporate public opinion into their lobbying strategies (Kellman, 1998).

Preferences of ordinary citizens are the bedrock of democracy and in influencing policy they play on decision makers in a variety of ways. Those who make policy are ". . . linked to . . . society by the flow of ideas between the two spheres" (S. R. Smith, 1995, p. 387). There is an intense interaction between ideas and institutions. The relationship between public opinion and government is dependent on the responsiveness of political leaders. In terms of national politics this responsiveness is most closely identified with the presidency and the Congress. Moreover, the influence of public opinion on governmental output has been the subject for perennial debate. Theories of democracy claiming that political leaders should be responsive to public opinion maintain that mass convictions should decisively bear on the decision-making process. There is clearly a difference between theory and practice.

Democratic policy-making mechanisms both react to and fashion preferences and opinions. Although the public has an influence on the making of public policy, the political attitudes and beliefs of ordinary citizens are not translated verbatim into policy outcomes. There are disjunctures between the preferences and values of the decision makers and those of the masses. In the American policy-making process, public opinion does not dictate policy. Rather, it sets priorities for the public agenda. Its impact on the formulation of actual policy is somewhat more restricted. In the health care arena the influence of public opinion varies, depending on its nature and that of the specific policy issue (Jacobs, 1993; Jacobs & Shapiro, 1995).

When public opinion is vigorous and enduring, it impacts on agenda setting, the process by which an issue moves to the forefront of policy discussion, and is assigned a high priority by officials in the executive and legislative branches of government. For example, in the Clinton presidency, health care reform was placed high on the public agenda because public opinion so desired. Issues not assigned significance by public opinion afford policy makers more discretion in their actions. The scope of public opinion is also of importance. It can be general or more specific in nature. If it does not focus on details, such as those related to administrative structures, decision makers again enjoy more latitude in this regard. Public opinion will exert less influence in situations when it is uninterested or uncertain and when an issue is not salient. In these circumstances policy makers usually yield to specific interest groups. On the other hand, if public opinion strongly supports a policy, decision makers will challenge particular interest groups. Although the public does not dictate public policy, it guides governmental output and can and does affect certain phases of the policy-making process. As noted above, it influences agenda setting, interest-group leverage over policy makers, and the making of detailed administrative arrangements. One study revealed that two-thirds of governmental output corresponded with the wishes of public opinion. The same correspondence was found when changes in public opinion were related to policy changes at various levels of government (Greenberg & Page, 1993; Jacobs, 1993). Thus, it is important that nurses contribute to societal dialogue via the discussion of candidates and issues.

Given their propensity to vote, it was expected that respondents to the survey would have participated in organized political campaigns in some way. Also of importance is the fact that the ANA promotes the political awareness and education of nurses. Its political-education program encourages nurses to become involved in political campaigns and teaches them how to do so. Furthermore, its structure includes a Department of Governmental Affairs whose principal purpose is to involve nurses in the political process. Its staff emphasizes the significance of political activism for every nurse. Yet, well over a majority of the sample (56%) never canvassed and campaigned for candidates. Political activism would help with the general public perception of nursing.

Political parties need funds to fight election campaigns, to maintain viable interelection organizations and to provide research facilities and other assistance for their leadership and elected public officials at various levels of government. In the United States elections and campaigns are expensive and are becoming a permanent feature of political life. The era of permanent campaigns has arrived. Money, their lifeblood, has a big role in the making of public policy through its financing of political persuasion. Given America's "hi-tech" political arena, campaign costs have increased steadily and rapidly. Election campaigns are financed by contributions from individuals, political parties, the candidates themselves, and political action committees. The largest portion of electoral funds is derived from individual contributions (Alexander, 1998). This is especially true in the case of presidential nomination finance. Federal matching funds and bank loans guaranteed by these funds are directly related to such contributions. As far as congressional campaigns are concerned, it is noteworthy that in the 1996 election cycle individual contributions accounted for nearly 67% of the cost of Senate races and over 50% of the amount needed for contests in the House of Representatives. Although, as previously noted, the turnout for presidential and midterm elections has declined since the 1960s, the number of political donors has increased. In fact, the base of electoral contributions in the United States is quite large (Brown, Powell, & Wilcox, 1995; Hrebenar et al., 1999; Shields & Goidel, 2000).

From the individual perspective, these contributions represent a considerable commitment. People donate for a variety of reasons. They might want to advance a specific cause or aid the efforts of a specific political party, its candidates or some faction of the party in a bid for power. They might identify with a particular wing of the party or believe that if the party and/or a specific candidate is victorious, either national or personal benefits will be realized. Many contributors have goals that they hope will result in political, legislative, judicial or administrative action. They will make a donation hoping that the appropriate individual will assume a position of authority in government, thus securing favorable governmental output. Then there are goals that are extraneous to the particular party or candidate. People contribute out of a sense of responsibility, feelings of patriotism, obligation, friendship with a political figure, belief in a two-party system or even ego satisfaction or exhibitionism (Alexander, 1972). Fifteen percent of the respondents to the survey indicated they always contribute money to support candidates. Seventeen percent usually did so. Forty-two percent contributed occasionally and 27% did not become financially involved. In the sample by far the tendency was to contribute occasionally.

One strategy to increase nursing's influence in the political arena is to aid nurses in their pursuit of leadership positions. One would anticipate that nurses would financially support their colleagues who run for public office. However, many nurse political candidates report that contributions of money and time from their peers are scarce, even though they contested an election as nurses and for the purpose of giving nursing another public voice. One such contestant was disturbed by the naivete of a number of colleagues who believed that if she lost her first race, she could always run again. To this she rightly responded: "Someone who is first time out and loses, is out" (Canavan, 1996b, p. 13). This pattern was confirmed in interviews undertaken by this author with nurse candidates.

A significant development in American electoral politics over the course of the last twenty-five years or so is the growth of political action committees (PACs) as an important part of financing electoral campaigns. PACs are a major force in the political arena with the potential to affect electoral results as well as public policy. These units are conduits through which organizations raise and distribute funds for the purpose of influencing the nomination and/or election of favored candidates for public office. More specifically, a PAC is ". . . a political arm organized by a corporation, labor union, trade association, professional, agrarian, ideological or issue group to support candidates for elective office . . ."(Alexander, 1998, p. iii). PACs solicit voluntary contributions that are then consolidated into larger, more meaningful amounts and donated to favored candidates or political party committees. These organizations provide a means for groups to participate in electioneering. As of 1999 there were 3,798 PACs (Edwards et al., 2000). During the 1995–1996 election cycle, 2,091 PACs contributed $5,000 or more to congressional candidates and they accounted for over 98% of all PAC contributions to federal contests for public office (Zuckerman, 1998).

Operating at the federal and state levels of government are two types of PACs: the affiliated and the independent. The former kind is created by an existing organization as a separate unit. Sponsored by corporations, trade unions, or trade associations, for example, these PACs are connected to a structure that is able to supply financial resources to pay administrative and fundraising expenditures. Independent PACs, on the other hand, are freestanding. Being officially autonomous and independent of any association, they must pay their own administrative and fundraising costs out of the funds they raise. These PACs usually focus on a specific issue or are aligned with a particular ideology.

Each type has its advantages and disadvantages. Not having to be concerned with raising sufficient funds to cover their costs, the affiliated PACs must restrict their solicitations to a tightly defined pool of potential donors. Corporate-sponsored PACs can solicit donations from executives, shareholders and their families. In a similar vein, labor-sponsored PACs and those of trade associations must limit their potential pool of donors to members and their families. On the other hand, PACs of the independent variety, having to raise money for their operating and fundraising activities, can solicit contributions from the public at large (Zuckerman, 1998). Although PACs have always been with us in one form or another, their massive growth was a response to reformist campaign finance legislation following the

Watergate scandals in the early 1970s that restricted the behavior of profit and nonprofit organizations in the political arena.

Nursing organizations, such as the ANA and many of its components, have PACs. Realizing that nursing had no internal structure to effectively penetrate the political system, and recognizing the impact of the AMA's political activism, in 1971 a small group of nurses from New York State established Nurses for Political Action, a national organization separate from the ANA and the state nursing associations. Its creation afforded the profession a potent instrument to reward or punish legislators through the provision of funds and the sharing of voting records with constituents. It was hoped that with its new unit nursing would become ". . . a national, viable force in changing the health care delivery system" (Rothberg, 1985, p. 134). Although this organization caused concern in national and state nursing associations, its importance was recognized. It served as a forerunner to the ANA's political action committee that was established in 1974 as the Nurses' Coalition for Action in Politics. With its birth political consciousness raising for nurses had a new instrument. At a later date it was renamed ANA-PAC. The purpose of this organization is to:

> promote the improvement of the health care delivery system by raising funds from State Nurses Association . . . members and contributing to the support of candidates— financially with volunteers, and other campaign activities—for Federal office who believe and have demonstrated their commitment to the legislative objectives of the American Nurses Association. ("ANA-PAC Endorsements," 1996, p. 7)

It is quite probable that a part of the sample that made political contributions gave them to the ANA-PAC or PACs of other nursing organizations.

The ANA-PAC has experienced tremendous growth. In the first part of the last decade it showed a greater increase in contributions than any other single PAC. Its donor base increased from 6,000 to 22,600 participating nurses, and in 1998, contributions for the third consecutive year surpassed the one-million-dollar mark ("ANA Opposes," 1996; "ANA-PAC Tops," 1999; "Health Care Reform,"

1994). Financial resources result from numerous small donations rather than a few large ones. To encourage participation and show appreciation, those nurses who donate $250 or more receive recognition at a special annual luncheon at the House of Delegates. Moreover, there are special benefits for those individuals who contribute over $500.

Elections provide a means whereby interest groups can turn their economic power into political power. PACs funnel vast sums of money to political campaigns. Their role in presidential nomination finance is not as central as in the case of congressional campaign finance. The percentage of congressional campaign funds contributed by PACs has increased steadily since 1972, reaching its zenith in 1988 in terms of proportion of funds provided (43% for House contests and 26% for senatorial campaigns). Since that date the share of PAC-generated monies has decreased. In 1998 it registered 35% and 18% for the House and Senate respectively (Brown et al., 1995; Hrebenar et al., 1999). Contributions from individuals remain the single largest source of political funds.

PACs flex their political muscles with campaign contributions in the hope of achieving policy output favorable to their constituency. The ANA through its PAC is no exception. It provides nurses with the means for assuring an active role in the election of public officials. Except for policy making delegated to the administrative branch of government and the specialized policy making of the courts, public policy in the American political system is established by legislative enactment. Thus, interest groups focus a major portion of their efforts on the Congress.

They acquire important powers because of the PACs' ability to raise and aggregate money. The groups' political influence is enhanced without relationship to the number of members or the worth of their arguments. Also, groups can impose huge costs on the rest of the population (Stern, 1988). PACs can impact policy outcomes by influencing who holds a congressional seat. The effect of PAC campaign contributions on electoral outcomes is generally recognized. The ANA-PAC supported 270 congressional candidates in the 1996 election cycle, 252 in 1998, and 177 in 2000. Although it is not included in a list of the top ten PACs in the nation, it does rank high among those in the health care field. It is the thirtieth largest PAC in the United States out of more than 4,000. In the health care arena it is the fourth largest political action committee (*ANA 2000*, 2000; "ANA-PAC Fastest," 1995; "ANA-PAC Fundraising," 1996; "ANA-PAC Tops," 1999; "Political Update," 1998). The leader is the AMA's PAC, which is known as one of the biggest spenders in the political world and as an innovator in new methods of influencing political figures. For years it has been among the largest donors to political campaigns and having lost almost a third of its membership over the last three decades, its clout is disproportionate to its size. Not only does it outspend all other health care groups, but it disperses more money than PACs sponsored by larger, well-known interests such as the United Auto Workers, the National Education Association, and the National Rifle Association ("The Medical Profession," 1999; "The Top Ten PACs," 1996; Wolinsky & Brune, 1994).

Often the endorsements of a specific PAC show a preference for a particular political party. As in other cases, partisan identification is important to the ANA-PAC. Over time it has favored the Democratic Party. The 1998 congressional elections were no exception. Eighty-one percent of its endorsed candidates were Democrats and of these 88% were elected, an increase of 11% over the 1996 election, accounting for the PAC's best success rate ever (Canavan, 1996a). In the 2000 election cycle 82% of the ANA's endorsed candidates were Democrats and 87% of the candidates supported by the PAC were elected to Congress. This strategy of partisan attachment differs from that of the AMA, which does not place as much value on partisan affiliation or on agreement on issues. In the 1995–1996 election cycle it allotted 19% of its funds to Democrats (Edwards et al., 2000; "Nursing Supporters," 2000). One empirical study demonstrated that the AMA–PAC contributed more money to legislators who opposed the association's position on public health matters than it did to representatives who supported it (Wolinsky & Brune, 1994). Such action it was hoped would guarantee an open door. When the Clinton health care reform was being debated, the AMA–PAC swelled the campaign coffers of nearly every member of that Congress. This matter was ". . . the most heavily lobbied issue in the nation's history" (Seelye, 1994, p. A1) in terms of dollars spent and people engaged. The ANA was among the first groups of health care providers to endorse Clinton in his bid for the presidency. Such a strategy brought its reward in the form of twelve seats for nursing on the forty-seven-member professional advisory review committee to Hillary Clinton's health task force. The AMA received none. The political spotlight began to shine on the ANA with this endorsement and with the onset of the Clinton administration's health care initiative.

Reference must be made to the dearth of nurses in the United States Congress. Although nurses in government are not responsible for promoting the nursing position, being there to explain that position and respond to questions about the profession could be useful to legislative colleagues. This lack of representation impinges negatively on the profession. In the 1998 electoral cycle the ANA-PAC endorsed six nurse congressional candidates, including three incumbents. This group represented two percent of the endorsed candidates. Only the three Democratic incumbents were successful in the election. In the 2000 elections the ANA-PAC supported four nurses, three incumbents and one challenger. The three incumbents were re-elected and the challenger lost by a very slim margin. Congressional candidate is a relatively new role for nurses. In 1976 B. J. Kalisch and P. A. Kalisch observed:

> The nurse does not usually have the time, the energy, the available resources, the self-direction, the confidence, the assertiveness, or the will to move into active roles in our government. No nurse has ever been elected to Congress and . . . none have attempted such a challenge. (p. 29)

Most recently the ANA has made a concerted effort to increase the number of nurse congressional candidates.

Given the propensity of those already in office to win reelection, and not wanting to waste their money, the largest share of PAC contributions goes to incumbents. The ANA-PAC has followed this general trend. Of its endorsed candidates in the 1998 congressional election cycle, only 16% were nonincumbents. This percentage was significantly reduced to seven in the 2000 elections. Even when a PAC prefers a challenger, for practical reasons, it will often support the incumbent, who might even be hostile to its goals. It will not risk its money, if a district is not likely to reject its representative. Contributions to a challenger, if the challenger is defeated, jeopardize access to the political system. Electoral security is definitely important to the endorsement of candidates.

The governing body of the ANA-PAC, the board of trustees, in conjunction with the constituent associations, determines the endorsement of candidates for federal office (U.S. Congress and President). Following established criteria, the board screens candidates, endorses those friendly to the ANA's goals, and sets the level of financial and in-kind support to individual campaigns. Candidates for endorsement are recommended by various sources that include the constituent associations, the Nurses Strategic Action Team (N-STAT), the ANA's grassroots network of 50,000 nurse activists; the Senate Coordinators and Congressional District Coordinators, individuals who provide primary contacts with policy makers; ANA lobbyists and political staff; and even congressional candidates themselves. All nonincumbents are interviewed in their home congressional district as well as in Washington, D.C., the location of the ANA headquarters. When the board of trustees endorses a candidate for federal office, this endorsement is not official until it receives the approval of the candidate's constituency association. Having secured this, the endorsement is announced to the public. An effort is made to ensure that endorsed candidates have contact with nurses in their congressional districts.

PAC contributions to electoral campaigns affect policy output in ways other than helping to determine who gets elected to Congress. It is often argued that they are important because they provide access to those whom they have helped to win office. Thus, the purpose of these contributions is to buy access, not votes. Providing assurance that telephone calls will be returned and that the organization's point of view will be listened to and considered, they are viewed as an investment. One theory, based on an exchange model of influence, argues that legislators will grant access to an organization when it enjoys competitive advantage over its rivals in terms of their career goals (reelection) and when it is anticipated that the issues and circumstances responsible for this advantage will recur. There is a close relationship between issues and legislators' career goals. Interest groups such as the ANA must convince legislators that their cause will contribute to these goals. Obviously, organizations possessing the most resources championed by candidates are the most successful in this regard. Empirical research demonstrates that issue-specific associations impact on legislative behavior when career goals—that is, reelection—are not endangered. Frequently, electoral contributions help to garner support on issues that are not significant to legislators or their constituency (Conway, 1986; Mueller, 1993; R. A. Smith, 1995). In any case, access is important and it is not distributed equally. Groups that have abundant funds and are willing to invest them in political campaigns can enjoy greater opportunity.

Single-purpose organizations generally distribute funds differently in the two houses of Congress. This occurs because of differences between them. The bulk of the work in the lower chamber takes place in committees and that of the Senate is performed primarily by individuals. Thus, interest groups follow different rules in distributing funds across the two units. Whereas there is a close relationship between legislators' committee assignments and contributions in the House of Representatives, such is not the case in the Senate. A House member's contributions are based on committee membership. A senator's derive from party and voting record. There is a strong link between certain types of PACs and congressional committees, especially in the lower chamber. Some PACs go a step further. In addition to committee assignments, they value seniority or committee expertise. They realize that seniority on a committee courts advantages, such as additional power over the agenda and enhanced effectiveness in performing casework. Moreover, with long experience on a committee, a legislator gains expertise in a specific area and, with it, possibly additional influence over policy output (Grier & Munger, 1993; Romer & Snyder, 1994). Thus, in the House, especially in the health care arena, members' particular committees are targeted by PACs. In allocating contributions to committee members, a group may try to anticipate who the principal players will be on issues of importance to it.

When the Clinton health care reform was on the center of the political stage the largest donations went to members of committees that produced health care legislation. Citizen Action, a public interest group, reported that in the lower chamber, members of the Ways and Means and Energy and Commerce Committees received an average increase of $27,000. Colleagues not serving on health-related committees acquired only $3,000 more. In the Senate, Finance Committee members received the biggest contributions (Seelye, 1994).

In the Congress there are more actors in health care policy making than in any other sector. Each participant has a small, but frequently important part of the jurisdictional spoils. The scope and complexity of the policy area virtually guarantee that almost every committee will have a legitimate claim to some part of the action (Mann & Ornstein, 1995). Empirical longitudinal research focusing on the involvement of congressional committees in specific subject areas, such as agriculture or education, demonstrates that a greater range of these units deal with health care issues. Over time congressional responsibility for this area has proliferated. More actors have become involved. Jurisdictional responsibilities in the legislature reflect the growth in the size and complexity of the health care industry. Almost every committee in the lower chamber has held hearings related to health care. Comparing the fields of education and health care, it is noteworthy that whereas almost three-quarters of the hearings on the former topic have taken place in the single most relevant committee of the House, the committee with the most health care hearings has only approximately one-quarter of the annual total. The situation is similar in the case of the Senate. In a twelve-year period, four committees in the House and three in the Senate held more than a hundred hearings apiece on health care issues, indicating that this subject area has more congressional overseers than any other one. In the House intense activity took place in the Select Aging, Energy and Commerce, Veterans' Affairs, and Ways and Means Committees. In the Senate the Labor and Human Resources, Finance, and Select Aging Committees were the major players (Baumgartner & Talbert, 1995; Mueller, 1993). Given this situation, the PACs' appreciation of congressional committee composition and seniority is understandable. Many issue networks form around the activities of these units.

In the 1970s rule changes led to modifications in congressional organization that contributed to the proliferation of political power. Access became of increased importance to PACs. Traditionally, committee chairpersons and party leaders, exercising policy leadership, were in an especially good position to receive campaign donations because of their critical role in the legislative process. With the changes, full committees and their chairpeople lost power to a galaxy of subcommittees and a steadily growing professional staff that were needed because of the increasing complexity of the problems to be addressed. Moreover, changes in governance related to voting and amendment activity, among other things, increased the number of actors to whom PACs might appeal. More specifically, in the House the practice of referring legislation to more than one committee became quite common. In the Senate, norms that once preserved committee power disintegrated causing rampant legislative individualism and an aversion to consistent deference to committee recommendations. In addition, mechanisms were devised to supplement or even bypass the standing committees. Points of access were multiplied with the devolution of authority (C. L. Evans, 1995; Petracca, 1992) and, thus, PACs assumed a different role.

Throughout the 1980s more modifications in the political environment, but especially the fact that two Republican presidents opted not to involve themselves in depth in domestic policy, again increased the number of congressional points from which to launch policy. In the American political system, given shortcomings resulting from fragmentation of the policy-making responsibility, localism and parochialism, seniority in legislative committee assignments, and congressional scrutiny of administration, executive leadership has been critical to legislative policy making. Lacking the tools to provide the necessary coordination of a legislative program, congressional leaders turned to the President for leadership in policy making.

The enormous range of presidential activity permits the White House to have a significant role in various phases of the policy-making process, such as agenda setting. It is the chief executive's responsibility ". . . to mobilize the broad coalitions necessary to enact legislation in a heterogeneous policy network and the larger legislative process . . ." (Peterson, 1993, pp. 430–431). Thus, interest groups do not restrict their activities to the legislative branch of government and presidents incorporate favorable interest groups into their legislative coalitions. Presidential involvement with interest groups is operationalized by interest-group liaison strategy. One dimension of this technique focuses on the amplitude of the relationships to be cultivated with the interest-group universe for purposes in general and for specific policy domains. Thus, interactions are either exclusive or inclusive. Another important facet of the strategy relates to the substantive focus of relations with interest groups, which is either programmatic or representational. Interest-group liaison strategies serve a variety of distinct presidential purposes: legitimization, the building of consensus, outreach or representation, and partisan coalition building. Changes in the political arena and in presidential needs dictate adjustments in liaison techniques (Peterson, 1992).

Thus, all interests, and in this case nursing interests, should be prepared at all times to react to a new policy-making environment.

When presidential leadership was absent, the situation was ripe for policy entrepreneurs, ". . . the authors and promoters of particular approaches to reform, who help define the issues of the debate" (Peterson, 1993, pp. 430–431). In this role career goals and advancement are tied to an effort to realize major policy endeavors. Just as an economic entrepreneur invests capital in an idea to realize a profit, a policy entrepreneur invests political capital in an issue to reap benefits. These people did not emerge from the traditional sources of policy initiatives: committees and subcommittees. Their forums included investigative subcommittees, special committees, and ad hoc groups in Congress. It is noteworthy that legislators as well as professional staff are identified with the role of policy entrepreneur. In addition to being in elected or appointed positions, policy entrepreneurs may also be external to government in interest groups or research organizations. These folks seek to gain visibility and establish themselves as specialists of value and initiators of innovative policies (Kingdon, 1995; Mueller, 1993).

When Newt Gingrich became Speaker of the House in 1995, other changes took place. There was a reversal in the direction of the power flow. He created a centralized decision-making structure with himself at the apex. He ruled with a firm hand, selecting committee and subcommittee chairpersons on his own, rather than by a vote of the Republican Conference, a partisan organ. He also made it quite clear that these officers could be removed at any time. Obviously, they and others did not enjoy the same latitude as in the past (Serafini, 1995). This new situation had connotations for PACs in terms of electoral engineering and access. It changed somewhat when Gingrich's ratings in the polls fell. With his image tarnished and his authority weakened, he gave committee chairpeople some latitude in agenda setting and promised to let legislation be first fashioned by committees. Today the speaker and heads of committees are stronger than they were two decades ago. Still the House of Representatives remains more disciplined and more centralized than the Senate where power is widely dispersed.

The effect of PACs on election results and legislative decision making has generated a great deal of debate. Researchers have studied the relationship between PAC contributions and legislative roll-call voting behavior. Some suggest that PAC funds affect legislators' support for legislation. Others conclude that such contributions do not exert a significant influence on roll-call votes. Unambiguous linkages between contributions and congressional voting have not been demonstrated. A review of the literature reveals that PAC contributions exert far less influence than is commonly believed (Conway, 1986; Evans, 1986; R. A. Smith, 1995).

Two alternative claims to the not-firmly-established vote-buying hypothesis have been advanced. One asserts that effects of PAC contributions are more likely to be witnessed in the confines of a committee than on the floor of the legislative chamber. The second affirms that the members' legislative involvement, not their votes, are most likely to be affected with PAC funds. Money does not buy votes. Rather, it mobilizes bias in congressional committee decision making. It buys the members' time, energy and legislative resources that committee participation requires. In general, interest groups and their financial arms have little, if any, influence on roll-call decisions (Hall & Wayman, 1990; R. A. Smith, 1995). Hall and Wayman contend:

[G]roups allocate their various resources (1) to mobilize strong supporters not only in House committees but also on the Senate floor, in dealing with executive agencies, and in various other decision-making forums relevant to the group's interests; (2) to demobilize strong opponents; and (3) to effect the support of swing legislators. (pp. 814–815)

Voting is related to a galaxy of factors, only one of which is campaign contributions. Some others, such as party identification, incumbency, constituency characteristics, constituency–representative relations, the interest-group constellation, the administration's position that is important for members of the president's party, personal conceptions of good public policy, cues from congressional colleagues, and a member's own policy attitudes must be taken into consideration (Kingdon, 1989). Whether campaign contributions affect votes is a function of a number of factors. It takes more than money for an interest group to secure a favorable vote on an issue.

This discussion has focused on activities of PACs in general and, specifically, the ANA-PAC at the national level of government. It is noteworthy that the use of PACs in the states has been as significant as that at the national level. Many state nurses' associations have a PAC that is active in subnational politics and operates in a fashion similar to that of the units involved in national politics. Typical is the PAC of the New York State Nurses Association (NYSNA-PAC). Nurses throughout the state take part in the endorsement process by providing the NYSNA-PAC names and dossiers of candidates worthy of support. The dossiers include information such as correspondence, newspaper articles, and campaign materials related to their positions on health care policy. Candidates are then requested to fill out a questionnaire and some are interviewed by nurses residing in their constituency. If the candidate happens to be an incumbent, NYSNA-PAC will examine the individual's voting record on health care issues and sponsorship of legislation.

The governing body of the NYSNA-PAC makes recommendations for the endorsement of candidates that are forwarded to NYSNA's board of directors for final approval. There are various types of endorsement, ranging from financial support or "in-kind" contributions to endorsements in name only. As at the national level of government, the purpose of such endorsements is to advance nursing's legislative agenda by fostering relationships with candidates. The latter's awareness of nurses' involvement and nursing issues is further enhanced by the fact that NYSNA members attend political fundraisers, make financial contributions to, and provide volunteer labor for campaigns ("Election Day 1996," 1996).

Given the behavior of the respondents to this survey concerning their participation in various facets of the election process, it can be concluded that, like the population at large, they shy away from what requires more effort in terms of time and money. They are prepared to vote and discuss candidates, acts necessitating little initiative and cooperation with others, but not to engage in those activities requiring more commitment and investment. In a pathbreaking study Milbrath and Goel (1977) compare voting to patriotism and label it a passive act. The respondents' behavior is interesting in light of the fact that 97% of them recognized the importance of political parties to the making of health policy decisions. Although professional associations and their PACs, and specifically, those affiliated with nursing, are heavily involved in extensive electoral politics, their message apparently has not been translated into widespread action by the sample.

Political competence, defined as the individual's perception of his or her ability to influence the formation of laws and policies, is an important element of any political culture. Beliefs pertaining to political competence have significant consequences for the operation of a political system. Thus, in an effort to ascertain opinions concerning individual political competence, those surveyed were asked to react to the following sentence: "People like me don't have any say about what the government does." This statement was overwhelmingly rejected. Ninety-five percent of the sample strongly disagreed or disagreed with it, indicating a belief that influence can be used. This finding contrasts with previous studies (Hayes & Fritsch, 1988) that indicate nurses often feel powerless in terms of affecting change.

A facet of political competence relates to the strategies that are used in attempts to influence the decision-making process. Involvement, the hallmark of democracy, helps to define societal goals and provides legitimacy to the political system. It can take many forms, including the various electoral strategies previously discussed. Other modes of participation, such as communal activity and networking, may be added to the list. These activities, which often lack a partisan focus, take place, for the most part, outside the electoral arena.

Participants in this survey were thus presented with a list of activities and asked to identify those in which they had engaged to influence the development of health care policy. The list included: (a) contact local and county elected government officials; (b) call or write government agencies involved in establishing health care policy; (c) attend official public meetings; (d) contact media—newspapers, radio, TV; (e) contact elected state or federal officials; (f) contact other individual or group, such as _____, (specify); (g) contact political party organization(s); (h) petition; (i) demonstrate/protest (implied as peacefully); (j) unionize; (k) strike. Fifteen percent of the respondents "sat on their hands," so to speak, in that they had never undertaken any of the activities. A majority failed to engage in seven of the 11 activities. They had never contacted the media (58%), worked with other individuals or groups (74%) or political party organizations (85%). Significant numbers were not involved with petition drives (51%), demonstrations or protests (75%), unions (85%), or strikes (94%). On the other hand, a majority of the respondents— 78%, 78%, 72%, and 69% respectively—had contacted local and county elected government officials, called or written governmental agencies involved in establishing health care policy, contacted state or federal officials, and attended official public meetings. Engagement in these activities is congruent with respondents' strong endorsement (95%) of the notion that an effective role in policy development requires communication with public officials. A higher percentage of the participants in this study (72%) had contact with a state or national official than those in the ANA's "Speak Up" market research panel survey (60%). The national association uses the panel to gather information related to the profession ("Speak Up," 1994). Given that American political norms encourage direct citizen contact with elected representatives, these high percentages are not surprising. Moreover, these activities constitute the normal paths suggested by the nursing literature, especially in textbooks, and by professional associations in the field. Often the latter organize letter-writing and postcard campaigns, sometimes with a prepared message, targeting officials and agencies at various levels of government. As in the case of participation in the electoral arena, the sample selected less demanding activities.

To compare the activities that they had engaged in with those they might undertake in the future, participants in the survey were then asked to identify how they would act if they wanted to be active in the development of health policy. In responding, they were to refer to the aforementioned list of activities. The preference order for future consideration duplicated and even magnified the results of the previous question. Of interest is the fact that, for a first choice, no one selected contact with a political party, petition, demonstrate/protest (implied peacefully), unionize, or strike. In fact, no one chose the last two activities and the percentage of respondents who designated the first three as second and third choices was minuscule (under one percent). For all practical purposes, these strategies were ignored. The 1960s witnessed the rise of protest and various forms of direct action, including strikes, marches, demonstrations and sit-ins, which supplement traditional lobbying techniques. Protest or subtle forms of disobedience, ranging from attending a protest meeting to participating in a protest demonstration or boycott, can be effective tools for citizen participation in policy making.

The media has always demonstrated a willingness to cover the unusual. The protest-media-politics triad has a special significance.

There is an interplay between these three elements in creating and communicating issues and in affecting public policy. News coverage is essential to the success of protests, but their relation to institutionalized politics impacts on the news media's response to them. Thus, these nontraditional or unorthodox tactics could be worthwhile. Catching the attention of the media, protest forms, and conflictive framing of issues promote publicity of a particular cause or message, expose the public to issues it might not otherwise encounter, and influence public policy and politics. Moreover, direct action can be effective in transmitting preferences to public officials. This is especially true concerning preferences about specific policy initiatives. The triadic relation between political processes, protest and the news media merits recognition (Oliver & Maney, 2000).

The National Labor Relations Act of 1935 gave employees the right to organize in labor organizations and to engage in collective bargaining. Within twelve years, with the passage of the Taft-Hartley Act in 1947, employees of nonprofit hospitals and health agencies were stripped of these rights. Nurses working in such facilities were consequently exempted from contract negotiations and their earnings and working conditions declined significantly in comparison to those of other professional and nonprofessional groups. It was only in 1974 that the Health Care Amendment to the National Labor Relations Act restored collective bargaining activities for employees in nonprofit health institutions. Thus, it was possible for nurses in all sites of employment to join unions. The passage of this amendment was a great victory for the profession. Following a resolution supported by the House of Delegates in 1956, the ANA, arguing that nurses were receiving substandard wages, for eighteen years actively lobbied in favor of the amendment that revolutionized nursing as well as unionism (McCullough, 1995). Scores of health care professionals swelled the ranks of trade unions that were no longer the exclusive property of blue-collar workers. Many labor organizations fervently competed for the sympathies of nurses.

Unionization and collective bargaining have been controversial issues within nursing because of its long history as a profession of dedication, altruism, self-sacrifice, and service as well as the correlation between nursing and a religious calling. The crucial questions are whether trade unionism is compatible with nursing professionalism and whether or not collective bargaining can be regarded as a professional endeavor. Numerous reasons have been cited for the incompatibility of these elements. First and foremost, it is argued that a profession is not a trade. Trade unionism is believed to taint the profession and to rob it of the autonomy needed to interact with the many constituencies nursing confronts. There are many unions competing for the representation of nurses, most of which consist primarily of blue-collar nonprofessional workers. Composed of and controlled by non-nurses, trade unions are seen as inappropriate units to represent professional nurses, given that the issues of economic security and professional practice are so inextricably related. Beletz (1985a) affirms:

> Trade union representation destroys nurses' unique professional identity and renders them pawns designated to provide the adrenalin for the economically hurting . . . trade union movement. Ultimately, trade unions are not protectors, but . . . predators of nurses' rights and this, therefore renders trade unionism incompatible with nursing professionalism. (p. 147)

Conceived as a divisive force, trade unionism, according to its nursing opponents, at best decreases and, at worst, completely destroys the profession's power. Not only does it create discourse for the profession, but it confuses the public. In essence, joining a union means relinquishing rights to control all aspects of professional affairs, the hallmark of a profession. For this camp, trade unions represent a barrier to nursing's drive for governance.

This group notes that workers substituting for nurses may perceive the professional nursing license as a barrier. This is important to labor organizations representing scores of unlicensed health care workers. This license promotes the job interests and economic rewards of these nonlicensed members. By controlling the professional nurse, the union controls the key to the salary structures for most hospital personnel. Moreover, such control affords an opportunity for the expansion of the roles of nonprofessional nursing personnel and thus reduces the wage differentials between the two types of employees. And then, nursing opponents of trade unionism are quick to point out, there is less need to employ a professional, if the role of the substitute worker is enlarged.

What organizing body should represent nurses has been a particularly delicate question. Believing that the professional organization will maintain a balanced perspective in its activities and have the interests of nursing at heart, many nurses supported the ANA in its effort to represent them through its Economic and General Welfare Program. Efforts toward collective bargaining commenced with members of the California Nurses Association during World War II but they were abandoned when the ANA refused to tolerate them. However, in 1946, after much discussion, the House of Delegates underscored the core value of promoting the economic and general welfare of nurses, which identifies with legislation securing the rights of nurses to organize and engage in collective bargaining, to protect their health and safety at their work site, and to eliminate the many faces of gender-based discrimination, among other elements. At this time the ANA assumed new responsibilities with the adoption of its economic security program, which endorsed state nurses' associations as exclusive representatives for their members in all matters affecting employment conditions and as their collective bargaining agents. This program, because of concern for the reputation of nursing, also included a no-strike clause. This policy restricted nurses' capacity to convince management to protect the mission of the profession for the public good. Coupled with the mandate of the Taft-Hartley Act, this stance delayed the growth of nursing's economic and general welfare program. The ANA eventually rescinded its eighteen-year-old no-strike policy in 1968. Nurses organized strikes, but frequently, rather than strike, they used tactics such as refusing to perform non-nursing tasks. Undoubtedly, the strike was perceived as a last resort.

A hallmark of the economic security program is its exclusive control by nurses representing themselves through the SNAs. Competition between the professional association and the trade unions for the authority to represent nurses was keen. Entering the field of labor relations, the ANA faced a formidable challenge. A former president articulated its message to its own constituency. She said:

> A paramount question facing the profession . . . is who will best represent nurses at the bargaining table? Will it be the truck drivers, meat-cutters, teachers, or nurses themselves? The answer of the ANA to this question has

been and continues to be that . . . it must be nurses who advance and control their own destiny. (cited in McCullough, 1995, p. 44)

Many nurses believe that the profession is best served by a nursing professional organization composed of and controlled by nurses.

In 1970 the ANA's Commission on Economic and General Welfare issued a strong statement that illustrated the connection between collective bargaining and professionalism. It read, "Nurses at all employment levels rightfully have the responsibility to participate in determining the terms and conditions of their employment and to share in decisions that affect the quality of nursing care they provide" (cited in McCullough, 1995, p. 44). This affirmation is stellar. Collective bargaining activities were to safeguard patient care and include the determination of standards for professional practice. Quality of patient care was to become a focal point of collective bargaining. Moreover, nurses were distinguished from other organized employees and their bargaining agents were differentiated from others. For the first time, employees and their representatives announced that they would protect the rights and interests of others, in this case the patients, at the bargaining table. In its early years the nursing profession's collective bargaining activities focused on remuneration. Now, often, wages are a secondary issue in negotiations. Emphasis has broadened to include a wide range of issues, such as contracts, services, practice matters, third-party reimbursement, comparable worth, patients rights, shared governance and safeguarding patient care against cost cutting, safe staffing and the quality of patient care, to cite a few. Many nurses believe that they have a right to a voice in these issues of critical importance to their performance. Typical of this belief is the following statement.

> We are not in this business out of charity, as altruists and Nightingalists would have us believe. We are here to make money, to use our minds and our skills, to provide services to patients on our terms. We need no longer apologize and feel guilty. (Ellis & Hartley, 1995, p. 317)

Of the 2.2 million nurses working in health care, approximately 350,000 have joined unions (Freudenheim & Villarosa, 2001).

Although the ANA is proud of its very successful Economic and General Welfare Program, which stresses protection of the rights of nurses to organize and bargain collectively, the collective bargaining activities of the SNAs generated philosophical conflicts concerning the advantages and risks of professional association bargaining. As noted previously, for many nurses professional values are not compatible with collective bargaining. A nationwide poll commissioned by the ANA in 1991 revealed that 67% of the registered nurses surveyed accept the concept of collective bargaining (Fuller-Jonap, 1994). Still the issue of compatibility continues to nag the profession, even though it has been vehemently argued and demonstrated that when substantial and unambiguous affirmation of professional values is included in a contract, unionization and professionalism are compatible (Fuller-Jonap, 1994; Zerwekh & Claborn, 1994). Moreover, it has been shown that there is a congruence in the definition of a professional in the National Labor Relations Act and in the sociological literature.

The ANA structure reflects this dichotomy in opinion. In terms of support for unionization, collective bargaining for professional nurses is usually found in states identified with significant union activity. Twenty-five SNAs adopted collective bargaining as a professional practice advocacy tool and the rest championed workplace advocacy. The former, partly in response to raids by other unions, formed the State Nurses Association Labor Coalition to create and implement a national labor agenda for registered nurses. In addition, the ANA created a committee on professional practice advocacy in reaction to the appeals of the other set of SNAs. The hope was that structural changes, resulting from the efforts of these groups, would accommodate the needs of both camps, each representing the interests of professional nurses within the framework of the association.

The coalition's efforts bore fruit. The United American Nurses (UAN) was created at the 1999 House of Delegates with the scope of enhancing nurses' access to collective bargaining through the ANA, reinforcing the labor program of the ANA and its constituents, and creating an effective national labor agenda. Speaking at the founding National Labor Assembly of the UAN, Linda J. Stierle, Executive Director and Chief Executive Officer of the ANA, claimed: ". . . We want nurses to be represented by nurses at the institutional, state and national levels through an autonomous labor body, which will establish and implement a progressive ambitious national labor agenda, as well as develop labor policy for [the] ANA" (*ANA 2000*, 2000). Membership is voluntary and limited to SNAs involved in collective bargaining activities. Associate membership is available to constituent members of the ANA whose bylaws provide for a collective bargaining program, but who do not presently represent nurses in this capacity. Moreover, the new entity is an insulated body, meaning that SNA members in management positions cannot participate in the UAN or exercise any decision-making authority in relation to it. In terms of its stand on labor issues, the UAN is autonomous and it advises the ANA on the implications of proposed policies for labor. ANA executive staff is responsible for the implementation of UAN programs. Structural arrangements of the new organization include a governing body, the National Labor Assembly, and an Executive Council, an organ to act on behalf of the membership between meetings of the governing body. The group recently affiliated with the American Federation of Labor and Congress of Industrial Organizations (AFL-CIO) to gain its support in labor disputes and to decrease conflict with its unions attempting to organize nurses.

The birth of the UAN is a milestone. It is the largest American nurses' union, over 100,000 strong with nurses from 23 states, and the only national union that commits all of its resources to the support of nursing. It offers advantages to the ANA, from a membership perspective, in terms of both recruitment and retention because it makes it possible to serve professionals searching for significant collective bargaining support. Many constituent associations, already having organized nurses, have provided an easy target for membership raids by other labor unions. Also, trade unions, growing their nursing membership, have been able to challenge the SNA as the professional representative. At the national and international levels, the ANA's authority as the voice for nursing has also been under pressure. The UAN confronts these problems. It strengthens the ANA and reinforces the SNAs' labor programs. It provides stronger fortification from attacks and threats. In addition, the financial implications must not be overlooked. The UAN has the potential to raise funds in addition to ANA membership dues ("National Labor Entity: United American Nurses," 2000). The challenges of this young organization are many. Of top priority is unity, a theme that plagues many facets of the profession. Exemplifying the enhanced activity of nurses' unions, at the start of 2001 the Massachusetts Nurses Association withdrew from the ANA, claiming it was too moderate. Earlier the California Nurses Association had become independent and signed an agreement with the United Steelworkers of America.

The ANA has not only attempted to meet the needs of those who identify with collective bargaining strategies, it has created different arrangements to ensure access to effective workplace advocacy for those practitioners not interested in collective bargaining. It is the responsibility of the Task Force on Professional Practice Advocacy to serve this constituency and to amplify work underway designed to support SNAs identified with workplace advocacy, which includes education, lobbying, and advocating singly and collectively to advance nursing's agenda. More specifically, this task force focuses on the structure and amplification of ANA support of SNAs so that all nurses will experience safe work environments, job security and a role in decision making concerned with patient care. Thus, SNAs can separate their ANA connection from union activities. The concern that a direct union connection might impinge negatively on lobbying efforts and other professional activities is no longer a threat. If SNAs have no interest in collective bargaining, because the UAN is a separate entity within the ANA, they can avoid identification with it.

These recent organizational changes, the UAN and the Task Force on Professional Practice Advocacy, represent attempts to unite the ranks of professional nurses. In the words of ANA President Beverly L. Malone: ". . . we have built a house that has room for all nurses, regardless of specialty, job title, or where they live or practice" ("ANA Creates New 'House'," 1999, pp. 1). Although there have been modifications in structure and attitude related to trade unionism, it is too early to make any judgments.

Given their behavior and preferences for action, it is clear that the sample is not a champion of trade unionism or collective bargaining. But at the same time, it is noteworthy that 53% of the respondents strongly agreed with the notion that the ANA and the SNAs should actively pursue legislation supporting the economic welfare of nurses. Thirty-three percent simply agreed with this idea. This phenomenon can be interpreted in different ways. It could be that there is a difference between the respondents' beliefs and actions or between theory and practice. Respondents to the survey might believe in the economic welfare program of nurses, but fail to engage in or support activities affiliated with it. Another explanation focuses on tactics. It could be that respondents accept economic welfare as an objective, but rather than pursuing it through trade unionism and collective bargaining, they favor the legislative path. They might be of the belief that economic welfare is to be secured through the legislative process.

Until the mid-1970s, demonstrations were the most prevalent form of job action among nurses. Mass demonstrations were used as well. The strike was not given a great deal of consideration as a weapon to be used frequently. In fact, in the hope of achieving favorable working conditions for the nursing profession, the ANA announced that nurses had voluntarily relinquished the right to strike. Although the professional association prohibited strikes, many of its members did not oppose them. A higher incidence of strikes occurred, particularly after 1969, indicating a growing militancy that persists today. Landmark strikes by California nurses took place in 1966 and 1974. In the first one nurses resigned in mass during a disagreement over salary demands. In its endorsement of the strike as an instrument for attaining economic objectives, the SNA not only broke with the policy of the national organization, but with tradition as well. Eight years later, nurses undertook a strike when contract negotiations failed in San Francisco. This strike, which was supported by the ANA, attracted national attention and it centered interest on matters related to collective bargaining with health care agencies. Strikes by nurses are no longer a rarity. Attitudes toward them have changed as militancy has increased. Now the ANA condemns strikebreakers. Most recently it has offered strong support to strikers in New York State and in Massachusetts.

Although nurses use the strike and the ANA rescinded its no-strike policy, it must be remembered that this instrument is formally regulated by national and state law. Thus, there is much variance in its use. Strikes have achieved positive results for the profession and they have also indicated why their general use is problematic. For example, some strikes have shown that nurses have not had the powerful allies and clout needed to achieve their professional goals. More specifically, they do not always enjoy support from other sectors, especially physicians and the public, two potentially powerful allies. Supervisory members of the nursing profession might be prohibited from striking by law, or be of the opinion that job action is incompatible with professionalism, or they might side with management. They cannot be counted on for support. Other hospital employees, another potential pool of allies, constitute a rival constituency. These are the people whose work makes nurses' work redundant. With the absence of nurses, their importance is enhanced. Thus, their support is not automatic nor is that of other health care unions. Unless a monopoly over a critical service already exists, most likely strikes will not contribute to the attainment of professional goals. Strikers might discredit their claims and even themselves (Levi, 1980). Involving many uncertainties, use of the strike must be given careful consideration.

Often there is a dichotomy in professional groups between elites and mass subdivisions that may identify with different rules and different clienteles. The use of appropriate tactics has served as a basis for such a division within nursing. The conflict is between nurses who are engaged in administration, education and research—that is, the leadership—and those working in service. This schism reflects the cleavage between leaders and followers evident in any political culture or community. The first constituency favors pressure and lobbying activity, whereas the second prefers collective action, including strikes. This dichotomy creates a sense of defensiveness in both camps. Given their preferences, respondents to the survey, discarding the option to strike, reflect this division. This dichotomy also has another ramification. Although both camps pursue professional status, the achievement of greater control over decisions affecting patient care in the hospital setting is more important to clinicians, thus creating further conflict with nursing's leadership (Beletz, 1985b; Davies, 1995; Levi, 1980).

Responses relating to strategies engaged in and to those that might be used to influence the decision-making process indicate a preference to act on an individual basis. In terms of first, second and third choices of strategies to impact policy development, only two percent, four percent, and six percent, respectively, of the sample opted to contact other individuals or groups. Respondents were asked to specify the sources they would contact. Indicating "other health care groups" or "other nursing groups" most of the responses were generic.

Communal or group activities, of which there are many different types, account for another participation mode. This type of political action has become more popular worldwide. Involving communication and group efforts to confront community, social, and other kinds of problems, this mode of involvement requires a great deal of political sophistication and initiative. Occurring outside the electoral setting, it lacks structure and partisan focus. Participants determine their own framework of participation including the agenda, strategies, and timetable. Having such control, those who take part in communal activity have more opportunities than those whose participation is restricted to political campaigns. They can provide more information and employ more political influence. As opposed to other participation modes, communal activity places control of participation with the group and, therefore, enhances its political influence.

Empirical research has demonstrated that Americans have exhibited a propensity to participate in this type of political action. In fact, public life in the United States has long been rooted in voluntary membership groups (Skocpol, Ganz, & Munson, 2000). Currently a major intellectual debate focuses on the nature of social capital, that galaxy of associations, clubs, and grassroots communities at the foundation of American society. On the one hand, it is argued that within the last thirty years more than a third of the civic infrastructure has evaporated leaving Americans, in the words of Putnam (2000), "to bowl alone." On the other hand, critics of this position assert that social capital is not dead, but merely experiencing a major modification. Older associations and networks are being replaced with a myriad of smaller ones, many of which have a grassroots orientation. In other words, all community is local (Dionne, 1998; Ladd, 1999). Both camps provide empirical data to support their argument.

The strongest predictor of participation in communal activities is education. Age, gender, political party affiliation and union membership have less impact on this participation mode than others (Dalton, 1996). Given that the better educated are significantly more likely to participate in this strategy, it was expected that it would be appreciated by the sample. Such was not the case as indicated by the statistics cited above. In practice, the respondents' identification with communal activity was less than that of the general public. Once again, they are not group oriented and their actions belie their beliefs. A significant portion of the sample (92%) affirmed that nurses and nursing organizations should develop coalitions with other groups to strengthen nursing's role in policy development. Power is acquired through pacts with others and the groups with which nurses might form alliances are as diverse as the topics about which they are concerned. The galaxy of coalitions in which the ANA participates confirms this fact.

Intra- and extra-professional strategic alliances are necessary for the long-term success of the professional association. When interest groups find common interests on which they can join, they increase the probability of finding a correspondence between the policy they want and the underlying attitudes of the proximate policy makers to whom they must appeal. Organized nursing has created interdisciplinary coalitions at all levels of government to advance its agenda. It has aligned with organizations that share goals, have leverage, and have complementary and necessary resources. These coalitions, according to Wilsford (1991) are critical

> [B]ecause the lobby, lobby, lobby system is a complex combination of constraints and opportunities and requires a presence simultaneously in multiple arenas. Constraints include delay and incrementalism in policymaking. Opportunities come from the numerous alternative arenas available. But the number of arenas also constrains, for it often requires political action in more than one arena at once. Alliances between interest groups and policy makers at all levels of the administration and of Congress provide not only indispensable access into the policymaking process for the groups but also provide policymakers with the support they need in their conflicts with each other. . . . (p. 234)

Organized nursing understands that coalitions are vital to the success of an association, given the nature of the previously discussed issue network. Often the more alliances with which a group is affiliated the better. Organizations might be in a coalition on one issue and adversaries on another. Coalitional lobbying has become a keystone of American politics. Interest groups relate to others with similar goals, but not to their adversaries. If there is communication with opposing organizations, it happens through a chain of other groups or a liaison or emissary and not directly. In the health policy domain interests choose their allies, for the most part, within their own organizational categories. External groups, such as labor unions or the various citizens' organizations, are often considered adversaries. However, they are selected as allies more frequently than in other domains. Consequently, the health domain is not as rancorous as others (Heinz, Laumann, Salisbury, & Nelson, 1990; Salisbury et al., 1987). The development of broad policy alliances and the grassroots approach incorporating informal groups are important keys to success.

Many of the requisites for participation in communal activities are held by nurses and many of the procedures involved are well known to them. A participant, like a nurse making a nursing diagnosis, gathers information related to a particular concern and compiles it in clear and concise fashion. An analysis is then prepared and, as in the planning stage of the nursing process, a decision is made about what will be done with this information, how it will be used and how it will be distributed. Just as a nurse shares data with other professionals, information is offered to colleagues and other groups (McIntosh, 1989).

Furthermore, this individual orientation manifested by nurse educators and also the clinicians in another study with which this author was identified (Delevan & Koff, 1990), is not congruent with the realities of the nursing profession. Lowery-Palmer (1982) observes:

> Ideally nurses place great emphasis on the individual. . . .
> In reality, however, because nursing work is defined in terms of complex organizational structures, the nurse is responsible for groups of patients and groups of co-workers [sic] and is accountable to groups of doctors and groups of administrators . . . the nurses' work primarily involves an interpersonal or intergroup process. (p. 194)

It is surprising that this group alignment does not carry over to nurses' perception of the political arena, which also emphasizes "groupness." Moreover, the effectiveness of an occupation is not measured by individual efforts alone. The efforts of all its members must be considered. Thus, an occupation's public image consists of individual and collective elements. Furthermore, ". . . [T]he goals of an occupation are only in a limited sense individual, for the individual responsibility of practitioners and consciousness of the aims of the occupation are very much a function of collective action" (Vollmer & Mills, 1966, p. 158).

It is important to realize that groups are significant actors in diverse political endeavors. Having come to exert greater influence on the political stage, group campaigns are often indistinguishable from those run by political parties or the candidates. The sample failed to realize that effectiveness of a profession is not gauged by individual efforts alone and that power derives from identifications cultivated within and external to the profession.

Responses concerned with strategies that could be employed to influence the development of health policy indicate that participants in the survey do not understand the complexities and penetrating nature of a postindustrial and mass society. Given their preference to act alone or on an individual basis, it is evident that they do not recognize the difficulties affiliated with the realization of desires in the political arena and the crucial need for communal activity with many diverse organizations, including those related to health care and otherwise. The importance of creating multifaceted or interdisciplinary alliances was not appreciated. The informal aspects of politics, which often are just as important as the formal aspects, were not recognized. Moreover, respondents were not especially interested in enlisting support from the informal face-to-face network of social groups—family, peers, workplace acquaintances, and so on—which are effective mechanisms of interest articulation.

In addition to slighting group action, as noted above, the sample does not view contact with political parties as being important to policy development, even though an overwhelming majority was of the opinion that decisions concerning health policy in general and specifically the nursing profession are made along political party lines. Brief reference must be made to the role of both entities in the policy-making process. In the American political system the relationship between interest groups and political parties has changed over time. Interest groups, extending their range of activities, have become major actors and thus the influence of political parties has eroded. The battleground for the competition between the two entities is provided by electoral campaigns. Political parties at one time completely controlled these contests, but in the 1950s, with the rise of candidate-focused campaigns, they began to lose their command. The increase in the number of interest groups and their reliance on modern technology caused parties to lose even more control over diverse types of campaigns, ranging from those whose purpose is to elect a candidate to those designed to sell a particular policy to the public (Hrebenar et al., 1999).

Also, it is generally acknowledged that, to a large degree, interest groups and political parties are mutually exclusive. Groups experience difficulty in achieving and maintaining influence in states with strong political parties. On the other hand, organized groups flourish and reap benefits in states with a weak political party system (Gitelson, Conway, & Feigert, 1984; Huckshorn, 1984). Nurses wanting to impact policy development should bear this consideration in mind. Moreover, they should recognize the importance of communal action. It is imperative that options be kept open so that either parties or groups, depending on the particular situation, may be utilized. Also, it must be remembered that in a competitive political party system voters are able to influence specific policies.

The importance of keeping options open cannot be overemphasized, given that most recently the politics of access and influence have been drastically modified. The new subsystem politics are characterized by openness, increased complexity, and greater competitiveness. The fluidity of issue networks must also be appreciated. In this environment the individual action preferred by the respondents to this survey is no longer appropriate. The development of broad policy alliances and utilization of groups, both formal and informal, are important keys to success.

The ANA actively pursues disparate alliances and courts both political parties by enjoying a high profile and making its presence felt at the Republican and Democratic Conventions. At these gatherings with other health care organizations and non–health care groups such as the AFL-CIO, it has cohosted receptions to honor Congressional dignitaries as well as popular hospitality suites, women's and patient safety rallies, and domestic-policy forums, focusing on a wide variety of subject areas ranging from health care and education to the environment and crime. In addition, it has hosted luncheons for nurse delegates, alternates to the Convention, and other "friends of nursing" in attendance. Wanting to be a strong and visible bipartisan organization, the ANA consistently networks at these gatherings.

If problems related to meeting the needs of the public and the nursing profession are to be addressed effectively, a multifaceted effort is crucial. All of the actors in the health care system—personnel, decision makers including third-party payers, and consumers—must be involved in the dialogue. Major issues involve the amalgamation of political, bureaucratic, professional, and consumer interests. Broad participation is a prerequisite for progress and change.

Another surprising finding related to strategies and policy development is the priority assigned to the media by respondents to the survey. In terms of the activities engaged in to influence the development of health care policy, contact with the media ranked sixth. As for strategies to be utilized, if one wanted to influence health care policy, it ranked next to last with two, six, and 11% choosing it as a first, second and third choice respectively. The expanding political and electoral role of the mass media was not recognized by the sample. This result contrasts with that of another study in which this author participated that focused on a cross section of nursing positions. In it, respondents demonstrated a willingness to use the media for purposes of access to the political system and the public (Delevan & Koff, 1990).

It is critical that information get to as diversified an audience as possible. An important component of this audience consists of journalists. Their significance derives from the fact that in passing information to others, they help shape their understandings. Mass media affirm widely held beliefs, values, and stereotypes, and serve as agents of socialization. They alert the public and key decision makers to developments and potential developments related to their interests. Moreover, the principal health care actors rely on the media as sources of information about what their colleagues are doing or might do and about insights into the perceptions, concerns, and expectations of various constituencies. Many instruments of the media with a large audience have reporters specializing in health care. Despite this, of note is the outcome of the Woodhull study on nursing and the media commissioned by Sigma Theta Tau. It concluded that nurses and the profession are significantly overlooked in the media's coverage of the health care scene ("Nurses Missing," 1998).

The worth of a news item depends on whether it directly or indirectly affects large numbers of people and in what ways. Given the broad scope and dynamic nature of health care, it has great potential for news worthiness. Kaplan and Goldberg (1997) assert:

Readers and viewers look to journalists, in print and on the air, for more than late-breaking news. They look to journalists for reliable and clear guidance about what the latest developments may mean for their health, their finances, and in some cases, their professional lives and strategies. (p. 107)

The value and importance of the media cannot be neglected, although its influence on the process and content of public policies depends on the nature of the issue, the stage of the policy-making process, the time frame and the political and media systems (Paletz, 1998).

Many opinions held by the public originate from images of nurses portrayed by the media. It is important to note that to a large extent it has portrayed the nursing profession in a negative manner. Nursing roles have often taken the form of a gender-based social identity and nurses have been typically presented as "go-fers" for physicians or as promiscuous sex objects. Despite the fact that their dedication to their work is supposedly of a religious nature, in the media they are frequently open to suspicion regarding morality in their social relationships. The media is more gentle and inclusive in its treatment of physicians. A reversal of this attitude toward nursing is related to a change in the role and position of women in the social system. Nowhere was the degradation of the nursing profession more clearly manifested than in the television series "Nightingales." The press has also contributed to this negative contemporary image. For example, one content analysis of newspapers revealed that community health nurses are depicted as traditional, passive, and restoration-oriented providers, whereas previously they were described as being progressive, innovative, influential and prevention-oriented (Deloughery & Gebbie, 1975; Iglehart, 1987; Kelly & Joel, 1995; Krantzler, 1986; Milio, 1985). The media has not been, nor is it always, a friend of the nursing profession.

Depending on which aspect of a nurse's activities is being focused on, a nurse is thought of as a slave or an angel. In activities that are carried out in conjunction with a physician, the nurse is often depicted as a slave or drudge. Possessing less sophisticated technical skills, this practitioner's authority is inferior to that of the doctor. On the other hand, when the nurse uses expressive talents and caring is the important function, this figure becomes the ministering angel. In spite of negative exposures, some surveys indicate that nurses are positively received by the public. For example, polls have shown that a large segment of the public would be willing to have advanced practice nurses assume some of the functions performed by physicians and that nurses are competent and caring (Kelly & Joel, 1996).

In an effort to erase the effects of the negative and unrealistic portrayal of nursing, the Tri-Council for Nursing created Nurses of America, a national, multimedia undertaking designed to inform the public of nursing's real role in the health care delivery system. Affiliated with this endeavor is a publication entitled *Media Watch*. Other projects also promoted nurses in the media and prepared them to interact with it to foster public understanding of the profession. These efforts included the National Commission on Nursing Implementation Project, a vehicle to raise public awareness of nursing's role. To this end, materials defining health care needs and trends as well as the contribution of nurses to health care were prepared to serve as a basis for dialogue between the profession and the public it serves (*The Nation's Nurses*, 1988).

The public's perception of nursing and how it is practiced affects recruitment to the profession. The image projected by the media determines, in part, who will want to become a nurse. If a career is devalued in the media, its prestige decreases and, in turn, practitioners command less respect as knowledgeable professionals. A positive media image is critical to a profession from another perspective. The extent of its influence in the political arena and the respect and importance assigned to political figures by the profession are determined by each group's perception of the other. This view, in part, is generated by the media. Mass media have stimulated significant public discourse about professions and, thus, have changed the strategies professions use to articulate their claims.

Also it is noteworthy that in terms of the development of health care policy, respondents assigned more importance to contact with local and county government officials than to those at the state and national levels of government. The same holds for those activities they engaged in to influence policy development. The significance of "grassroots" power is not congruent with the realities of the professional life of nursing or health care delivery. State governments play an important role as a result of their regulatory powers. They exert control over both the institutions in which nurses are educated and in which they practice. Moreover, their financial authority and powers concerning licensure and credentialing, delivery of service, and third-party payers are significant.

Respondents were not in accord with the present allocation of responsibility for the planning and delivery of health services. Their prevalent belief was that it should be at the national (33%) level of government. Next priority was assigned to state government (29%) followed by local (14%) and county (9%) governments and the rest of the sample favored the private sector or some mix of governmental responsibility. Moreover, as might be expected, a significant percentage of the sample (98%) thought that nursing should be represented on all major local, state and national bodies that recommend, establish, or implement health care policy. Such representation frequently has not been achieved.

There has been much discussion of the relative roles of health care professionals and consumers in developing health care policy. Some people say that the planning and control of health care policy decisions should be primarily driven by members of the health professions. Others argue that the people who use health services should have more say in these decisions. Believing that these choices should be made equally by health professionals and the people who use their services, a majority of the sample (58%) had an opinion that can be placed in the middle of this continuum. Thirty-five percent assigned more responsibility to health professionals and six percent attributed more importance to the people who use health services. The majority opinion assigned more weight to the public than present arrangements in the health care delivery sector.

A crucial part of the rules of the political game in the United States is federalism, signifying a division of power between the national and state governments. Although federalism is an ancient concept, as it exists today, it is largely an American invention. In this arrangement the relationship between the central or federal government and the state units may be characterized as coordinate. With limitations on the powers of both levels of government, both are subordinate to the Constitution. Most nations have a unitary form of government, meaning that all or most of the power is lodged in the center. Subnational units exist, but at the whim of the center. Thus, they have a subordinate relationship with the national government. Federalism affects many different facets of American politics, including the public policy decision-making process. Policy is determined both in the states and at the national level of government. This affords American citizens greater opportunity to participate in policy making than their counterparts in many other nations.

Recognizing that people can be active in federal and state policy developments, a section of the questionnaire was designed to elicit the respondents' levels of political cognition and political participation in each sector. Those surveyed were given a series of federal and state legislative and regulatory initiatives in the health care field and they were asked to identify their awareness and role in seeking the passage or defeat of them (unaware of the legislation, aware but took no action, active involvement). In addition, they were asked to indicate their personal position (support or oppose) on each item. Federal projects cited included the Health Security Act, Health Professions Education Extension Amendments, Reauthorization of Agency for Health Care Policy and Research, Family and Medical Leave Act, Extension of Home Health Services under Medicare, and Medicare and Medicaid Reimbursement for Advanced Practice Nurses. With the exception of the continued federal funding and reauthorization of the Agency for Health Care Policy and Research, now known as the Agency for Healthcare Research and Quality, the majority of the sample was aware of policy actions. In all cases, with this one exception, awareness prevailed over unawareness. In that the survey was administered to academics who are supposed to be heavily involved with research, and that this particular agency is identified with significant research efforts and support related to nursing, it is somewhat surprising that the majority was unaware of this reauthorization. Created in the late 1980s, the Agency for Health Care Policy and Research has been primarily concerned with research related to the quality and effectiveness of health care services, the development of practice guidelines and the assessment of technology. Nursing pervades all of its initiatives. This is another indication of the profession falling short in terms of identification with research endeavors.

However, in general, the political cognition of the sample as it relates to policy development at the federal level of government was high. It is significant that in the cases in which the majority of respondents was particularly aware of legislative initiatives, there was very little active involvement in the issue, such as letter writing, or direct communication with public officials and other influential actors in the policy process. In individual cases the percentages for active involvement, for the most part, did not come close to those for awareness. In all instances the no-action category was greater than the active involvement one. When a minority of respondents chose to become involved, involvement was greatest with reference to the Health Security Act, Medicare and Medicaid Reimbursement for Advanced Practice Nurses, and the Health Professions Education Extension Amendments in that order.

Individual support for the cited policy initiatives ranged from 79% to 99%, but in spite of this, nonaction prevailed. Personal opposition was highest in the case of the Health Security Act (21%) and relatively low in other cases, ranging from one to five percent. The former, enjoying the highest rate of opposition and the least personal support (79%), generated the most reaction. Active involvement on this matter, standing at 48% of the sample, far outstripped that for all other issues. This high degree of participation may be attributed to the extensive publicity given to the matter. Furthermore, many groups organized diverse types of intense campaigns related to the project. In spite of the sample's extensive participation on this issue, that of the previously mentioned "Speak Up" market research panels was somewhat higher at 56%. Opposition to the Clinton health reform plan was greater among members of these panels, ranking at 34% and support for it was less at 58% ("Speak Up," 1994). Rating second in terms of the respondents' participation (39%) was Medicare and Medicaid Reimbursement for Advanced Practice Nurses, a so-called "pocketbook issue," and in third place was the Health Professions Education Extension Amendments (31%). Involvement in other initiatives trailed far behind, ranging from 19% to five percent in the case of the reauthorization of the Agency for Health Care Policy and Research. It is noteworthy that these "pocketbook issues" enjoyed a higher level of participation among the "Speak Up" panelists.

The first two initiatives signified immediate and tremendous changes for the nursing profession. Thus, the high level of participation is understandable. The Health Security Act, if approved, would have meant a major transformation for the American health care delivery system and the providers of care. The Clinton Administration offered the reform in response to a galaxy of problems in the health care sector that included growing insecurity, increased complexity related to administration of the system, rising costs, decreasing quality, declining choices, and growing irresponsibility (White House Domestic Policy Council, n.d.). Rejecting the idea of a government-run health care delivery system, according to the project, services would remain in the private sector. The basis of the plan was managed competition, which involves ". . . using market forces to control health care costs and improve the system's performance" (Starr, 1994, p. 47). All Americans were to enjoy universal coverage and comprehensive health benefits reflecting mandated services. The reform specified a framework for the delivery of services that detailed standards and the comprehensive benefits the population was to receive. States and local communities were then free to tailor their own programs within the established parameters in an arrangement similar to the Canadian one. In this way they could serve their own needs as long as they conformed to the national guarantees and standards for quality and access to care. Essentially the federal government was to establish the foundation of the health care delivery system and then permit subnational communities to build on it as they wish. Having created the framework, the national government's role was to subside and allow the reformed private market to pave the way.

Each state and the bigger corporations were to have a large purchasing cooperative or health alliance whose task would be to organize the private market so that consumers would be provided with an array of private health plans from which they could make an intelligent and informed choice. Various groups of providers of health care services and insurers, in competition with one another, would prepare health care plans. The alliances and plans would negotiate and subscribers would be allowed to select from at least three alternatives that would include a health maintenance organization, other managed care plans, and a conventional insurance program. Promoting competition based on quality and price among the health plans, the health alliances were to organize the private market in such a way that consumers could compare the plans and make informed choices. The sponsors of the plans were to negotiate the benefits packages, conduct the annual enrollment, provide appropriate information to the consumer, and collect and disperse payments. They too were involved in managing competition. Competition was to be managed so that people would not be excluded from coverage because of their health status, and choice among the various plans was to be as easy as possible. Thus, managed competition was to have certain ground rules: open enrollment; standard, comprehensive benefits; accountability for quality of care; cost-conscious choice; and community rating premiums for consumers and risk-adjusting payments to plans (Starr, 1994).

The last three items require some explanation. With cost-conscious choice, government and employers make a fixed contribution to an insurance plan. Consumers benefit from the savings if a plan can offer the standardized coverage at a lower cost. On the other hand, if coverage is produced at a higher price, the purchaser assumes responsibility for the difference between the fixed contribution and the cost of the selected plan. Community rating underscores the equality of all citizens. It means that community-wide rates or the same premiums apply to all persons, regardless of their health status. Often health care plans attempt to attract the healthiest persons and avoid the sick. The incentive for such a practice is reduced with rate-adjusting payments, meaning that the sponsor's payments to the plan are based on the risk of the populations involved. Payments to plans attracting higher risk persons, for example the elderly or the sicker, are adjusted upward, whereas contributions to programs enrolling lower-risk people are adjusted downward (Starr, 1994).

In addition, the administrative arrangements of the health care delivery system were to be streamlined so that they would become more user friendly and, for the providers of care, more supportive and flexible. At the same time, unnecessary regulations were to be abolished. An improvement in the quality of care was at the core of the health security project. The various facets of performance were to be monitored on a regular basis. However, access to care, the appropriateness of care, outcomes of care, consumer satisfaction, health promotion, and disease prevention were to receive special attention. Research endeavors were to be emphasized and to have an important role in quality control. Soaring costs were to be restrained through the power of the competitive market, increased buying clout, lower administrative costs, caps on growth in expenditures for covered benefits, a limit in premium increases, and the reduction of health care fraud.

Financial resources for the plan were to derive from a variety of public and private sources. Employers were to pay 80% of the premiums and the employee the additional sum. For firms having under 50 workers, government subsidies would be available to aid employers in paying their share of the costs. The self-employed were to finance their own premiums up to an established amount and these costs were to be tax deductible. Government subsidies were to cover premium expenses for the unemployed and state and local governments were to support the costs for the poor. Medicaid, but not Medicare, was to be abolished. The federal government was to cover premium charges for retirees under the age of sixty-five. The financing of public-sector contributions to the cost of the health security program was to be inspired by the baseline concept, which involves the projection of expenses under current law and present trends. Having forecast federal spending increases, rather than merely finding more money to cover them, the Clinton proposal planned to utilize savings derived from programmed changes in federal health activities to cover new initiatives as they were being implemented. New revenues were to provide the remaining federal monies. These were to come from an increase in taxes on tobacco products, a one-percent assessment on the payrolls of large companies that have their own health alliances, and a partial recapture of savings to firms benefiting from lower health insurance costs for early retirees.

In short, the Health Security Act was based on the principles of security of coverage, simplicity, savings, quality, choice and responsibility. For the first time in American history, everyone was to take part in the solution of the American health care crisis and have a stake and role in the nation's health care and security. In closing his address in which he presented his health care reform to a joint session of Congress, President Clinton affirmed: "This is our chance. This is our journey. And when our work is done, we will know that we have answered the call of history and met the challenge of our time" (White House Domestic Policy Council, n.d., p. 106). However, this was not to be the nation's chance or the American people's journey. Furthermore, the call of history was not answered and the challenge of the age was not met. Comprehensive health care reform as outlined in the Health Security Act failed to secure congressional approval, confirming ". . . the conventional wisdom of how external forces (the president, public opinion, and interest groups) and internal conditions (committees, political parties, leaders, and rules and procedures) shape what Congress does" (Mann & Ornstein, 1995, p. 10).

This failure has been attributed to a variety of factors. When the plan was being discussed in 1994, the president was experiencing

difficulty with his own popular image and it is generally acknowledged that a weak president should not make strong demands on
Congress because of the likelihood of legislative inaction or stale-
mate. In addition, Clinton's reform proposal received tepid public
support because of its supposed identification with big government
and a strong bureaucracy, both of which are alien to the American
political tradition that features a basic distrust of government inter-
vention. Remaining deeply ambivalent about government, especially
at the federal level, Americans prefer private solutions to public problems. Moreover, the long time needed and the secret process that was
used to design the reform, plus its length and complex nature did not
aid in securing passage of the project. Economic factors were also important. At that particular time the American economy was boom-
ing and health care inflation had been curbed, at least for the
moment. This meant it was not as easy as it had been to highlight the
issue of rapidly increasing costs in the health care industry (Patel &
Rushefsky, 1995; Schick, 1995).

The press also contributed to the reform's failure. What reporters chose not to emphasize was as significant as the content they
featured. Moreover, they began to report a great deal on the reform
at an early stage of the decision-making process. As in an election
campaign, early press coverage rather than later reporting defines
key terms and sets forth alternative policy proposals. This tendency
is problematic for those people who begin to pay attention to politics at a later point in time. Jamieson and Cappella (1998) attribute
the public cynicism to this type of reporting. Furthermore, they note
that it depresses learning about issues, complicating public delibera-
tion in a period when the problems to be confronted are always
more complex.

In addition, with the Republicans in the Congress being united
in their opposition to the Clinton proposal and the Democrats in
both chambers being divided, partisanship was a problem. Given this
situation and the low level of public support for the bill, there was little incentive for negotiations to secure passage of the proposal. American institutional arrangements, manifesting the principles of the
separation of powers and checks and balances, also took their toll.
Many of these factors worked to the advantage of the powerful interest groups in the opposing camp. They were able to put together
an overwhelming campaign that confirmed the suspicion that in a

confrontation on a policy issue of importance, interest groups could strangle the power of a determined president and his political ammunition. The Health Security Act was not approved. As a result, the United States failed to join the ranks of a majority of the world's nations whose citizens enjoy universal access to the health care delivery system and universal coverage.

Nurses, as well as other professionals, have been persistent in their quest to obtain direct reimbursement for their services. This effort became especially evident in reference to legislation passed in 1983. It created a prospective payment system for Medicare recipients based on a classification that established pretreatment diagnosis categories for hospitals of 467 Diagnostic Related Groups (DRGs). In this framework patients are assigned to a DRG category based, for the most part, on their principal morbidity, treatment, age, and possible complications. Each DRG is linked to a specific number of days and cost for a hospital stay. If the patient is discharged early, the entire designated amount of reimbursement is kept by the hospital. On the other hand, if the patient is kept longer than the time allotted by the DRG category, the hospital is responsible for the additional costs. Some nurses felt that with the change to the new system, it was an appropriate moment to identify nursing services so that they could be differentiated from the general daily costs. Others developed methodologies to specify the acuity of nursing care so that these could be incorporated into the DRG classification. There have been many changes in this arrangement since its inception. Nursing has attempted to influence these modifications through its participation in decision-making structures, its efforts to cost out nursing services, and lobbying by major professional associations. Activities related to reimbursement for services are identified, for the most part, with advanced practice nursing which includes the roles of the clinical nurse specialist, nurse practitioner, nurse-midwife and nurse anesthetist.

Reimbursement efforts by nurses successfully penetrated the Medicare and eventually the Medicaid programs. In the case of the former, as of 1987, nursing services delivered in a Community Nursing Organization were reimbursable. These units, coordinated and managed by nurses, offer a package of Medicare benefits to the elderly in non-institutional settings. The package includes home care services; physical, occupational and speech-language therapies, medical equipment and supplies and ambulance services along with case management, health education and preventive services. In the same year certified nurse-midwives became eligible to receive payment from Medicare for their services, provided they worked in a Health Maintenance Organization. Two years after, certified nurse anesthetists, nurse practitioners, and clinical nurse specialists were authorized for Medicare reimbursement. Retribution depends on the location of service and the setting. Also it is usually related to percentage differentials for non-physician practitioner fees. This policy has been a bitter pill for the nursing profession to swallow. For example, it means that an advanced practice nurse performing a service can receive no more than 85 percent of the physician's charge for that same service. The rationale is that services provided by a physician supposedly differ from those offered by another practitioner. As long as reimbursement for advanced practice nursing is linked to physician reimbursement, the cost-effective benefit of advanced practice nurses will go primarily to physician practices rather than with society. As far as the Medicaid program is concerned, in all states there is mandatory reimbursement for care delivered by pediatric and family nurse practitioners and certified nurse-midwives. States exercise discretion for services provided by other advanced practice nurses. Federalism affects this program because coverage and reimbursement rates vary from state to state. The Federal Employee's Health Benefits Program and CHAMPUS, the arrangement for civilian employees and dependents of the military and military retirees, are other governmental programs that recognize the services of advanced practice nurses as being reimbursable. In addition, in many states advanced practice nurses enjoy third-party reimbursement by insurance companies.

This principle of reimbursement for services rendered involved a very intense and bitter struggle on the part of the nursing profession that still is not finished. Major opposition, as one might imagine, came from physicians who advocated remuneration only to the medical profession or for care requested by it. They argued that such a limitation on third-party reimbursement would aid cost containment efforts. In reality, the status and power position of doctors are reinforced and enhanced.

An analysis of the power distribution in the health care industry leads to the conclusion that financial independence is essential for any provider group that wishes to acquire power in the system . . . . The road to power for nurses and the road to third party reimbursement are one and the same . . . . (Maraldo, 1985, p. 71)

Members of the sample recognized the significance of fiscal autonomy in that 99% of them supported Medicare and Medicaid reimbursement for advanced practice nurses. In reality, however, the needs of the public and the influence of third parties reduce the health professionals' ability to set the conditions of their practice. Third parties are an important influence. They can stipulate the kind and method of payment as well as the type of care to be delivered. They control the mechanics of providing health care and serve to reduce health care providers' decision-making authority. In this particular instance, nurses as professionals were no different than any other constituency. The status quo is supported when a group's interests are in accord with it and when occupational interests differ from those of the so-called establishment, change is sought.

Respondents to the survey demonstrated less awareness of policies at the state level of government. More specifically, they were especially uncertain of general health care initiatives such as the state health plan, malpractice reform, and insurance reform, and more aware of issues more closely related to their profession, such as the regulation of nurses in advanced practice, prescriptive privileges for nurses, and third-party reimbursement for nurses. Interest was keener in the so-called "pocketbook" issues. It is precisely these issues that generated the most active involvement in the policy-making process. However, overall active involvement was slightly higher at the national level of government. As in the case of the latter, in all instances the percentage of those respondents who did not take action in reference to a particular policy was greater than that of those who did directly participate. There is a divergence between belief and fact. Although respondents to the survey were of the opinion that professional associations should have a strong role in policy development, they thought that individual nurses should have primary responsibility for influencing policy and that every nurse should take an active role in the development of policies favorable to nursing and the consumer.

Focusing on issues with personal financial implications has negative and positive connotations. On the positive side, as noted earlier, third-party reimbursement is important to the enhancement of nursing's image and power within the health care community. Part of nursing's inferior status, as noted, is due to the fact that the profession is not credited with being income producing. On the negative side, this particular issue has served as a source of further division within an already fragmented profession. The fact that advanced practice nurses are eligible for reimbursement in specialty areas of practice has generated hostility against this type of practitioner on the part of those colleagues not possessing this privilege. This and other related issues would be of concern to a large part of the sample because 44% of it was certified in an area of specialty practice. However, the gulf between advanced practice nurses and the rest of their colleagues impacts negatively on nursing's political efforts. As one nurse practitioner has observed:

> NPs [nurse practitioners] tend to be proactive, and nursing tends to be reactive. The biggest problem is that we have not been able to unify and say that what's good for NPs is good for nursing and what's good for nursing is good for NPs. ("25 Years Later," 1990, p. 16)

Such schisms weaken the profession's power in the policy-making process.

POLITICAL–LEGISLATIVE KNOWLEDGE BASE

In addition to knowing about participation in the development of public policy, it is important to understand how participants inform themselves about the issues involved. What efforts are made? What sources do they utilize and with what frequency? What is their access to pertinent information related to decision making? Answers to these questions determine how people conceive of, analyze, and understand public policies. Bearing this consideration in mind, a section of the survey instrument focused on published sources of policy related information. It listed a series of publications sponsored by professional nursing organizations (*The American Nurse, American Journal of Nursing, Capital Update*, the National League for Nursing's public policy bulletins, *Nursing and Health Care*, *Nursing Outlook*, the state nurses' association [SNA] newspaper and the American Association of Colleges of Nursing's newsletter), and official governmental sources (*Congressional Monitor*, *Congressional Record*, and the *Federal Register*), plus the *Chronicle of Higher Education*. Participants were asked about their familiarity with the resource (familiar, unfamiliar), their access to it (available, not readily available, obtained with added effort), and the frequency of use for policy content (frequently, occasionally, not at all).

As might be expected, the sample had greatest familiarity with nursing publications. By far the most familiar sources were the *American Journal of Nursing*, *Nursing Outlook*, *The American Nurse*, and *Nursing and Health Care*, which were known to 98%, 97%, 87%, and 82% of the sample respectively. *The American Journal of Nursing* is the oldest of the nursing periodicals and the official journal of the ANA. Founded in 1900, it served as a tool to unite members of the profession and as a means of education. Its uniqueness at that time was that it was controlled and owned by nursing professionals. Moreover, it linked the workers and the thinkers in the profession and allowed nurse educators, administrators and professional nurses in disparate work settings to engage in dialogue. Although it emphasizes the clinical practice of nursing, it contains a wide range of information related to public policy initiatives pertinent to nursing and health care at all levels of government, both national and international. Another ANA publication is the bimonthly, *The American Nurse*. Its objective is to keep its readers informed about changes in the nursing profession and in health care policy. Most recently it has expanded its editorial scope to include a larger variety of happenings in health care concerned with nursing and practice innovations, as well as human interest stories. Also, it covers extensively the activities of individual SNAs and the national organization. *Nursing Outlook* is published by the American Academy of Nursing. Although it focuses on current issues in nursing practice, education, and research, it also offers information on health policy developments and proposals that impact on the profession. *Nursing and Health Care* is the official journal of the National League for Nursing. Given the publisher's mission of promoting and monitoring effective nursing education and the academic basis of the survey's sample, it is not surprising that this journal enjoyed extensive familiarity.

Of the nursing sources, those most unfamiliar or least familiar to respondents to the questionnaire were *Capital Update*, the bimonthly American Association of Colleges of Nursing newsletter, the SNA newspaper, and the public policy bulletins issued by the National League for Nursing. These were unfamiliar to 41%, 36%, 27%, and 27% of the sample respectively. *Capital Update*, a legislative newsletter for nurses, is published twice a month by the ANA. As indicated by its name, it offers extensive coverage of the Washington scene, issues on the political stage, and ANA activities in this arena. It is an extremely useful source for those interested in concise statements of public policy related to nursing as well as the ANA's orientation on particular issues. For the most part, the last three mentioned publications are self-explanatory. They periodically update their readers on health care developments in their bailiwicks, as well as on general federal and state initiatives, and specific positions on public policy issues.

Of the non-nursing sources, the most familiar was the *Chronicle of Higher Education*, which was known to 80% of the respondents to the questionnaire. A weekly publication, as its name implies, it is devoted to all aspects of higher education. Its familiarity is understandable, given the sample's site of employment. In terms of familiarity, the official governmental sources were ranked as follows: *Congressional Record*, (64%), the *Federal Register*, (60%), and the *Congressional Monitor* (40%).

As far as nursing publications are concerned, *The American Nurse,* being cited by 47% of the sample, was by far the most popular source in terms of frequency of use for policy content. The closest competitors were *The American Journal of Nursing* and *Nursing and Health Care*, cited by 35% and 32% of the respondents to the survey respectively. They were followed by the SNA newspaper (27%), *Nursing Outlook* (24%), National League for Nursing public policy bulletin (20%), the ANA's *Capital Update* (20%), and the American Association of Colleges of Nursing newsletter (16%).

The sources used least frequently for their policy content were those issued by the government. The *Federal Register*, the *Congressional Record*, and the *Congressional Monitor* were cited as being used frequently by five, four and three percent of the sample, respectively. The *Chronicle of Higher Education* is in an intermediate category, being used frequently by 20% of the respondents to the questionnaire.

The government publications scored the highest in the category of sources not used at all. Of the nursing publications, the newsletter of the American Association of Colleges of Nursing held the same ranking. A majority (54%) of the sample claimed it never refers to this publication. This percentage plus the 36% of the respondents who indicated a lack of familiarity with this newsletter are noteworthy in light of the fact that the American Association of Colleges of Nursing was the most popular specialty organization for the sample in terms of membership. Also of interest was the high percentage of participants in the survey who never used the SNA newspaper (48%), the ANA's *Capital Update* (46%), and the National League for Nursing's public policy bulletins (42%), all of which are tailored to issues on the public agenda. This lack of familiarity and usage, especially in the first two cases, is understandable in light of the previously mentioned data concerning membership in the official voice of nursing. Many nurses are not members of the ANA and its affiliates. This trend is evident in the sample. Moreover, only a small percentage (5%) of the respondents to the questionnaire claimed to be active members of the National League for Nursing.

It would be logical to assume that there would be a close relationship between access to a published source of policy-related information and its frequency of use. Such was not the case. The highest percentage of the sample (47%) consulted *The American Nurse* frequently. However, responses to the survey indicated that it was readily available to only 12% of the sample. A majority (55%) claimed it was not readily available and 33% obtained it with added effort. In terms of being readily available, this publication ranked in tenth place out of twelve.

Nurse educators are responsible for making students aware of their potential to effect change and to empower themselves and their profession as well as the communities with which they identify (Batra, 1992; Galligan, 1985; Spradley & Allender, 1996). Thus, students require a comprehensive understanding of the health care delivery system and their role in it, the policy-making process as well as health care policies and issues in general, and specifically those pertaining to nursing. In addition, their political competence must be nurtured. In an endeavor to see how these matters were incorporated into nursing curricula, participants in the survey were asked to list the titles of courses taught into which such themes were integrated and to detail the specific content. It is noteworthy that 50% of the respondents did not deal with this subject area at all. Moreover, there was a dearth of whole courses devoted to this material.

Clinical and technical courses were cited by 80% of those who wove these topics into their classroom presentations. Leadership, administration, professional development and professional issues courses were noted by 27%. Nursing theory courses ranked third (11%). They were followed by courses focusing on health care delivery systems, social policy, and the politics of health care (9%); a miscellaneous category that included teaching practicum, senior seminar, research critique and interdisciplinary courses (7%) and ethics classes (3%). Tied for last place in the hierarchy (1%) were history of nursing and a category labeled "all courses." A clear distinction between graduate and undergraduate courses was not evident.

In terms of issues covered, the most cited focused on professional practice, social categories (elderly, homeless), and reimbursement for nurses. These were followed by health care delivery and reform, finance, insurance, access and availability, ethics, regulation, drugs and research, and education. Prevention and primary care and disease-oriented issues tied for last place. All of these issues are important. However, taught in bits and pieces the mission at hand is not accomplished. Also, with extensive emphasis on the first three categories, a balanced, proportioned, and comprehensive understanding of the policy-making process, health care policy and health care delivery, and nursing's role does not emerge. Conveying the importance of health policy, its major issues and the policy-making process is a significant challenge for nurse educators and to weave the subject matter throughout the curriculum is a difficult task that must be creatively and carefully planned.

It has been generally acknowledged that health policy materials have not been appropriately integrated into the nursing curriculum at the graduate or undergraduate levels (Batra, 1992; Leavitt, 1994). Thus, the situation in New York State is not atypical. Nursing education has not provided nurses with the tools to change the system, but rather to function in it. One respondent to the survey commented:

> Nurses are not taught "how to" become politically aware.
> For the profession to truly make an impression and have a
> strong political voice—on local, state and federal levels—

nurses need to be made politically aware. Ideally, this process would commence during nursing education.

More often than not, nurses have been socialized to a passive role rather than one for social action. Historically they have followed policies for which they have little, if any responsibility for developing. Nurses should understand the nature of the health care system and the policy arena to use both to their advantage. This is vital to advancing the interests of the profession. Otherwise others will make decisions for it.

The preparation of nurses for participation in the health policy-making process has received much attention in the professional literature (Buerhaus, 1992; Cohen, et al., 1996; Thomas & Shelton, 1994). Given the survey results, the matter perhaps has been addressed more effectively in the literature than in academia. Almost three decades ago, having a great deal of foresight, B. J. Kalisch and P. A. Kalisch (1976) warned:

> The benign neglect of political factors in the education of nurses fosters the omission of a critical element in understanding, planning and executing nursing services. A simple course in American government as part of a general education requirement is no substitute; nursing is unique insofar as applying the principles of politics is concerned, and a course in "politics of nursing" is desperately needed. . . . Student nurses will be increasingly involved in a political environment as they embark upon their professional careers. The ones who succeed will be the ones who learn to understand it, adjust to it, and turn it to the advantage of their profession. (p. 30)

These words are still cogent today. All institutions should have at least one course devoted solely to this subject matter. Moreover, it should have a historical dimension so that nurses with an understanding of the past will better comprehend contemporary issues confronting the profession. Curricular changes, at least in New York State, have not recognized this need.

A recent survey of changes in that state's nursing programs (Cohen, et al.,1997) reveals a concern with the clinical and practice environment. A political–legislative knowledge base is not reflected in curricula. There were additions or expansions of clinical sites in community and ambulatory settings, increased content on community-based nursing, and more emphasis on health promotion and illness prevention. The inclusion of policy making and health policy courses in the curriculum is important to the socialization of future members of the profession. Studies have underscored the need for this subject matter as well as its significance. Barry (1989) found that nurses involved in policy-making roles developed their political interest as a result of interaction with non-nursing elements after their formal nursing education had been completed. Hayes and Fritsch (1988) reported that nurses' political attitudes and political participation are enhanced by early political socialization and education. Hanley's work (1983, 1987) revealed the need for political education in all nursing programs. Her work identified this material as a predictor of participation in the policy-making arena. In a study by Archer and Goehner (1982), a significant percentage of the nurse leaders interviewed (94%) indicated they were not as politically involved as they could or should be. Low political participation was attributed to a lack of "know-how," meaning lack of knowledge of and skill in the political process. Other reasons were inadequate political socialization and education. It is evident that students, to avoid isolation from the arena where power games are played, must be aware of their role in the larger political system of which they are a part in addition to that within the nursing profession. As Milio (1989) stated: "The readiness of the profession for policy work in teaching, research, and the public arena has clearly arrived" (p. 318). This readiness is still present and awaits to be acted on.

The so-called "curriculum revolution" in nursing education suggests innovative changes in the integration of power, politics and public policy in the curriculum (Isherwood, 1995). However, nurse educators have been slow to embrace this movement. Its support is so small that the major question is whether it survives or not. Hesitation about acceptance may be due to nurse educators' belief that they themselves are not well versed in policy issues and lack this type of experience (Leavitt, 1994). The efforts of the New York State Nurses Association in this regard are stellar. It has endeavored to impress nurse educators with the importance of the legislative process and its impact on nursing practice and to prepare them for the incorporation of a political–legislative knowledge base into the curriculum. Given that education is the primary socialization agent for nurses, the lack of policy content and process in nursing curricula can cause students to ignore policy-related and political activities (Stimpson & Hanley, 1991).

In this chapter, mention has been made of disparate participation modes, all of which place diverse demands on the actors and have different outcomes. Each of the behaviors discussed is distinguished on the basis of the investment required in terms of the amount of initiative, effort, and cooperation with others. In their comportment, respondents to the survey demonstrated a preference for activities that demand, for the most part, lesser initiative, effort and time, and little collaboration with other individuals and groups. These choices have consequences for the type and amount of influence exerted and the scope of the outcomes. Activities, other than those preferred by the sample, are more effective. Also of importance to the outcomes of concern to nursing is the parochial and fragmented nature of classroom materials related to the political–legislative arena. Current course substance and role modeling by these nurse educators offer the future professional limited vistas, and, in all probability, much unrealized potential on the political stage.

Chapter 4

Conclusion

If nurse educators do not appropriately role model political behavior, can it be expected that members of the profession will participate in their professional organizations and in the political process? The study of political socialization agents explains a great deal about the way in which politics works and people behave. This volume has presented the importance of the political arena to the nursing profession. It has explored the role modeling behavior and attitudes toward political participation of a primary socialization agent: nurse educators. Cultural and social values, upheld by these academics, as well as their role modeling are among the essential features underlying the behavior of nurses on the political stage.

Participants in this study have an understanding of the importance of the political process to their profession and the need for a political role on the part of all professionals. However, at the same time, they have little inclination to perform that role and they do not provide positive role modeling in political activism. In this sample there is a dearth of role models whose behavior reflects the realities of the political process. Participation is thin in terms of the number of participants and the number of activities engaged in. These nurse educators have not taken advantage of the wide range of available power resources. They are wed to restricted patterns of interest articulation and goal achievement behaviors. Moreover, their actions are not congruent with their beliefs, which are one thing in theory and another in practice.

The results of this study might be used to explain in part nursing's status as a "sleeping giant" and its failure to realize its potential in the political arena, both of which have been lamented in the nursing literature for a long time. Professional socialization agents have evidently functioned in such a way that nurses have developed behavior appropriate to the clinical environment, but not to the political arena. This phenomenon affects these professionals as members or nonmembers of, and participants or nonparticipants in, professional associations; as potential agents of change in the health care and political systems; and as citizens.

As in all professions, politics pervades the nursing profession. It will determine its future and the form in which it survives as it has influenced its past. Nursing faces a more exposed and difficult situation today because it was not able to resolve its occupational and professional problems years ago when the environment was more conducive to its success. Competition in the political arena is and will become keener as the number of groups competing for shrinking rewards and resources increases. The profession will need to increase the number of politically active nurses to enhance its effectiveness on the political stage. The separation of nursing and politics is no longer accepted. Political activity is part of nurses' legitimate work. The professional voices of nursing affirm politics as a professional responsibility (Mason, 1990). The political context of nursing cannot be ignored.

Moreover, official sources, such as the Secretary's Commission on Nursing, a national advisory panel established by the United States Department of Health and Human Services, have recommended that nurses increase their participation in policy-making opportunities within the profession and at all levels of government (National Commission on Nursing, 1988). Other influential interdisciplinary bodies, such as the Pew Health Professions Commission, have concurred with this political thrust. In a report, the Commission (Pew Health Professions Commission, 1995) noted the need for health professionals to work with political forces. Furthermore, it affirmed, "The role of activist and advocate is not a new one for the health care professional, but it is one that must be recovered and forged anew. . . ." (p. xii).

Until recently most nursing politics have dealt primarily with nursing's own intraprofessional concerns. Although the profession has recognized the importance of the externalist dimension of power, and it has made great strides in exercising it, much remains to be done to further mobilize nursing into a significant political force. Results of this study indicate that the curriculum, role modeling, and mentoring are among the important instruments in this mobilization.

The curriculum is one of the major political socialization agents. Nurse leaders have related the deficits in the education of nurses in politics and public policy making to the profession's limited performance in the political arena (Stimpson & Hanley, 1991). Results of this study second the need for formal incorporation of a systematically developed political–public policy facet in already crowded nursing curricula and in continuing education activities. This is a difficult and delicate task. The nursing literature is rich with strategies to increase practitioners' understanding of and participation in public policy (Buerhaus, 1992; Diers, 1985; Leavitt, 1994; Martin, White, & Hansen, 1989; Sharp, Biggs, & Wakefield, 1991). Professionals, to assume a proactive stance, must be aware of, recognize, and understand current trends, issues, and questions to be debated. They must understand where, when, why, and how they will be discussed. Effective participation requires a comprehension of the politics involved. By understanding the political realities and the ways in which decisions are reached, nurses will be prepared to augment their power in health care and political arrangements. They will ". . . be able to understand the operation of the health care system from a broad economic, social, political, legal, systems and organizational perspective" as envisioned by the Pew Health Professions Commission (1995, p. xiv). Moreover, they will develop a unique perspective on their own profession and the communities they serve.

Politics, being concerned with who gets what, how, why, when, and where, focuses on power. However, in addition to being taught, power must be demonstrated. Throughout this work, reference has been made to the importance of role modeling. Within the educational system nurse educators are role models for nurses as well as for nursing students. Serving in this capacity, they are in a position to develop in others a commitment toward the profession that will create a concomitant obligation to a career and the willingness to assume a measure of individual responsibility and accountability for the advancement of the communities of which they are a part. Faculty members have a responsibility to demonstrate exercise of power through the projection of their community and interests. To develop an understanding of how to obtain and use power within the profession, in the workplace, and in other settings, nurses need a regiment of role models of appropriate and effective political participation.

Closely related to role modeling is mentoring, ". . . usually defined as a formal or informal relationship between an established older person and a younger one, wherein the older guides, counsels, and critiques the younger, teaching him or her survival and advancement in a particular field" (Kelly & Joel, 1996, pp. 297–298). There is a very thin dividing line between the two methodologies. A mentor can be and often serves as a role model. However, a principal difference between the two figures is that the former directly interacts with the other individual(s) in the relationship, while the latter does not necessarily do so. Moreover, whereas faculty and preceptor activities are time limited and specifically skill related, those of the mentor are not. This affords greater opportunity for the development of a multifaceted and long-term relationship with the mentor. Mentoring, a useful tool for the early enhancement of professional socialization, reinforces and complements role modeling, primarily because of its more personalized nature. Empirical research has demonstrated its significance (Archer & Goehner, 1982; Jonson, 1998).

These three instruments—curriculum, role modeling, and mentoring—taken together, are important to the exercise of professional power. They allow nurses to become aware of and familiar with the issues on the public agenda, to understand the political system and its operation, and to participate in it, hopefully with intelligence. Moreover, they combine the theoretical and practical aspects of learning with a personal touch that should motivate all participants in the educational endeavor to become more fully involved in the process of change.

Serious attention must be given to the political socialization of nurses so that new entrants to the profession will have a sense of political astuteness and an understanding of the basis of power. Nurses need to have more involvement in policy decisions affecting them. The results of this study would support the idea that a good place to start would be the universal enhancement of the curriculum, role modeling, and mentoring. Future members of the profession would be educated and encouraged to take responsibility for participation in the policy-making process. Education, in comparison to other socialization agents, is slow to bear fruit. Thus, time is of the essence.

Professional schools, through research, investigation, and employment of new knowledge, serve as agents of change. Nurse educators, as advocates and role models for students and nurses in general, are in an excellent position to nurture political awareness, advance the professional agenda, and forge change. Those whom they educate serve individuals, families and communities who can be mobilized to fashion the policies that make this service possible. Being responsible for preparing future professionals, nurse educators affect a significant number of people. Although their power is somewhat reduced in the workplace where clinicians tend to exercise more influence, in terms of interests and amount of power, academicians often have greater opportunity to affect the policy-making process (Tousijn, 2000). They have a strategic role in determining how the profession obtains, maintains, and employs the tools of power.

This research only begins to explore nurse educators' involvement in, their attitudes toward, and knowledge of the policy-making process. Implications can be drawn from this effort for possible faculty development, curricular enhancement and nature of the professional agenda. Being a project limited in geographical scope, this work must be considered a pilot study, hopefully to be followed by additional research based on diverse samples and geographic areas that would provide baseline and comparative data along with opportunities for generalizations related to the findings.

The American health care system is in a period of extreme fluctuation. In spite of its many accomplishments, there are significant deficiencies and discontent that have to be remedied. Actions at all levels of government are required. Nurses, as major providers of health care and the largest discipline among all health care providers, will be profoundly affected by any changes. As the profession searches for a new identity and a new role it must use the political arena to its advantage. The question is: will nurses collectively play an active role in the resolution of health care problems at all levels of government, or will they remain the "sleeping giant" in the health care industry? This is a critical question because, as noted throughout this work, the profession is becoming more and more shaped by political decisions. Nurses can be highly instrumental in bringing about a redirection of the health care delivery system. However, they must be prepared to fashion change and to be agents for this change. Above all, they and nurse educators, in particular, must not forget the advice of Florence Nightingale: "March! No system can endure that does not march " ("ANA '88," 1988, p. 977).

References

Abbott, A. (1988). *The system of professions: An essay on the division of expert labor.* Chicago: University of Chicago Press.

Alexander, H. E. (1972). *Political financing.* Minneapolis, MI: Burgess Publishing.

Alexander, H. E. (1998). The PAC phenomenon. In E. Zuckerman (Ed.), *The almanac of federal PACs: 1998–99* (pp. iii–v). Arlington, VA: Amward Publications.

American Medical Association: Power, purpose, and politics in organized medicine. (1954). *The Yale Law Journal, 63*(7), 938–1022.

American Nurses Association. (1965). *Educational preparation for nurse practitioners and assistants of nurses: A position paper.* New York: American Nurses Association.

American Nurses Association. (1991). *Bylaws as amended June 30, 1991.* n.p.: American Nurses Association.

American Nurses Association (2001). *New federal constituency fact sheet.* Retrieved July 17, 2001, from http://www.ana.org.

ANA at work. (1999, March/April). *The American Nurse.* Retrieved July 17, 2001, from http://www.nursingworld.org.

ANA creates new "house" for all nurses. (1999, July/August). *The American Nurse,* pp. 1,8.

ANA '88—pay us more and let us nurse—ANA's solution to the shortage. (1988). *American Journal of Nursing, 88,* 976–980.

ANA opposes the elimination of PACs. (1996). *Capitol Update, 14*(5), 2.

ANA takes poll of membership. (1996, October/November). *Report*, p. 12.

ANA 2000. (2000). Retrieved July 17, 2001, from http://www.nursing-world.org.

ANA-PAC endorsements. (1996). *Capitol Update, 14*(7), 7–8.

ANA-PAC fastest growing PAC in the U.S. (1995, June). *The American Nurse*, p. 9.

ANA-PAC fundraising report. (1996). *Capitol Update, 14*(23), 7.

ANA-PAC tops $1 million mark. (1999). *Capitol Update, 17*(1), 1.

Archer, S. E. (1982). Selected concepts fundamental to nurses' political activism. In S. E. Archer & P. A. Goehner (Eds.), *Nurses: A political force* (pp. 53–107). Monterey, CA: Wadsworth Health Sciences Division.

Archer, S. E., & Goehner, P. A. (Eds.). (1982). *Nurses: A political force.* Monterey, CA: Wadsworth Health Sciences Division.

Ashley, J. (1977). *Hospitals, paternalism and the role of the nurse.* New York: Teachers College Press.

Atkinson, P. (1985). The reproduction of the professional community. In R. Dingwall & P. Lewis (Eds.), *The sociology of the professions: Lawyers, doctors and others* (pp. 224–241). London: Macmillan Press.

Atkinson, P. (1993). The reproduction of the professional community. In R. Dingwall & P. Lewis (Eds.), *The sociology of the professions: Lawyers, doctors and others* (pp. 224–241). New York: St. Martin's Press.

Baer, E. D. (1987). "A cooperative venture" in pursuit of professional status: A research journal for nursing. *Nursing Research, 36*(1), 18–25.

Baim, O. G., Jr. (1972). Adult socialization. In *International encyclopedia of the social sciences* (Vols. 13–14, pp. 555–561). New York: Macmillan Company and Free Press.

Bandura, A. (1977). *Social learning theory.* Englewood Cliffs, NJ: Prentice Hall.

Bandura, A. (1986). *Social foundations of thought and action: A social cognitive theory.* Englewood Cliffs, NJ: Prentice Hall.

Barry, C. (1989). A descriptive study of the political socialization processes of nurses in specialized roles in federal and state governments. In *Dissertation Abstracts International.* (University Microfilms No. 89-19002).

Batra, C. (1992). Empowering for professional, political, and health policy involvement. *Nursing Outlook, 40*(4), 170–176.

Baumgartner, F. R., & Talbert, J. C. (1995). From setting a national agenda on health care to making decisions in Congress. *Journal of Health Politics, Policy and Law, 20*(2), 437–445.

Becher, T. (1990). Professional education in a comparative context. In R. Torstendahl & M. Burrage (Eds.), *The formation of professions: Knowledge, state and strategy* (pp. 134–150). London: SAGE Publications.

Beletz, E. E. (1985a). Games of power and politics: Trade unions and nurses' rights. In R. R. Wieczorek (Ed.), *Power, politics and policy in nursing* (pp. 137–148). New York: Springer Publishing Company.

Beletz, E. E. (1985b). Organized nurses and collective bargaining: Opinions, participation and militance. In R. R. Wieczorek (Ed.), *Power, politics and policy in nursing* (pp. 228–254). New York: Springer Publishing Company.

Bergman, R. (1985). Nurses as a social force. *Journal of Advanced Nursing, 10*, 197–198.

Berry, J. M. (1989). *The interest group society* (2nd ed.). Glenview, IL: Scott, Foresman/Little Brown.

Bertilsson, M. (1990). The welfare state, the professions and citizens. In R. Torstendahl & M. Burrage (Eds.), *The formation of professions: Knowledge, state and strategy* (pp. 114–133). London: SAGE Publications.

Blackwelder, J. K. (1997). *New hiring: The feminization of work in the United States, 1900–1995.* College Station: Texas A & M University Press.

Brante, T. (1999). Professional waves and state objectives: A macro-sociological model of the origin and development of continental professions illustrated by the case of Sweden. In I. Hellberg, M. Saks, & C. Benoit (Eds.), *Professional identities in transition: Cross-cultural dimensions* (pp. 61–81). Göteborg: Göteborg University.

Brewer, C. S., & Kovner, C. T. (2000). *A report on the supply and demand for registered nurses in New York State.* n.p.: New York State Nurses Association.

Brown, B., Nolan, P., & Crawford, P. (2000). Men in nursing: Ambivalence in care, gender and masculinity. *International History of Nursing Journal, 5*(3), 4–13.

Brown, C. W., Jr., Powell, L. W., & Wilcox, C. (1995). *Serious money: Fundraising and contributing in presidential nomination campaigns.* New York: Cambridge University Press.

Bucher, R., & Strauss, A. (1961). Professions in process. *American Journal of Sociology, 66*, 325–334.

Buerhaus, P. I. (1992). Teaching health care: Public policy. *Nursing and Health Care, 13*(6), 304–309.

Buerhaus, P. I., Staiger, D. O., & Auerbach, D. I. (2000). Implications of an aging registered nurse workforce. *Journal of the American Medical Association, 283*(22), 2948–2954.

Bullough, B. (1983). The relationship of nurse practice acts to professionalization of nursing. In N. L. Chaska (Ed.), *The nursing profession: A time to speak* (pp. 609–633). New York: McGraw-Hill.

Bullough, B. (1994). Nursing theory: History and critique. In B. Bullough & V. L. Bullough (Eds.), *Nursing issues for the nineties and beyond* (pp. 64–82). New York: Springer Publishing Company.

Bullough, B., & Bullough, V. L. (1994). Nursing organizations. In B. Bullough & V. L. Bullough (Eds.), *Nursing issues for the nineties and beyond* (pp. 22–31). New York: Springer Publishing Company.

Bullough, V. L. & Bullough, B. (1984). *History, trends and politics of nursing*. Norwalk, CT: Appleton-Century-Crofts.

Burau, V. (1999). The politics of internal boundaries: A comparative analysis of community nursing in Britain and Germany: Some preliminary observations. In I. Hellberg, M. Saks, & C. Benoit (Eds.), *Professional identities in transition: Cross-cultural dimensions* (pp. 239–253). Göteborg: Göteborg University.

Bureau of Health Professions. (2000a). *HRSA state health workforce profiles: New York*. Washington: U.S. Department of Health and Human Services.

Bureau of Health Professions. (2000b). *United States health workforce personnel: Factbook*. Washington: U.S. Department of Health and Human Services.

Burtt, K. (1998). Male nurses still face bias. *American Journal of Nursing, 98*(9), 64–65.

Canavan, K. (1996a, November/December). ANA-PAC scores impressive number of wins. *The American Nurse*, p. 16.

Canavan, K. (1996b, April/May). Nurse ranks grow in legislative bodies nationwide. *The American Nurse*, p. 13.

Capuzzi, C. (1980). Power and interest groups: A study of the ANA and AMA. *Nursing Outlook, 28*(8), 478–482.

Carnegie, M. E. (1994). The evolution of organized nursing. In O. L. Strickland & D. J. Fishman (Eds.), *Nursing issues in the 1990s* (pp. 13–21). Albany, NY: Delmar Publishers.

Carr-Saunders, A. M., & Wilson, P. A. (1933). *The professions*. Oxford: Clarendon Press.

Castro, F. W. (1999). After the wave: The welfare state professionals in Swe-den. In I. Hellberg, M. Saks, & C. Benoit (Eds.), *Professional identi-ties in transition:Cross-cultural dimensions* (pp. 43–59). Göteborg: Göteborg University.

Code, L. (1988). Feminist theory. In S. Burt, L. Code, & L. Dorney (Eds.), *Changing patterns: Women in Canada*. Toronto: McClelland and Stewart.

Cohen, B. J., Levin, R. F., Bashoff, M. L., Ellis, E., Condie, V., & Gelfand, G. (1997). Educators' responses to changes in the health care system. *Journal of the New York State Nurses Association, 28*(2), 4–7.

Cohen, S. S., Mason, D. J., Kovner, C., Leavitt, J. K., Pulcini, J., & Sochal-ski, J. (1996). Stages of nursing's political development: Where we've been and where we ought to go. *Nursing Outlook, 44,* 232–237.

Collins, R. (1990). Changing conceptions in the sociology of the professions. In R. Torstendahl & M. Burrage (Eds.), *The formation of profes-sions: Knowledge, state and strategy* (pp. 11–23). London: SAGE Publications.

Conway, M. M. (1986). PACs and congressional elections in the 1980s. In A. J. Cigler & B. A. Loomis (Eds.), *Interest group politics* (2nd ed.). (pp. 70–90). Washington: CQ Press.

Creason, N. (1978). Registration and voting participation of four faculty groups. *Nursing Research, 27*(5), 325–327.

Crompton, R. (1987). Gender, status and professionalism. *Sociology, 21,* 413–428.

Cutting, D. W. (1982). Lobbying. In S. E. Archer & P. A. Goehner (Eds.), *Nurses: A political force* (pp. 173–194). Monterey, CA: Wadsworth Health Sciences Division.

Dalme, F. (1983). Nursing students and the development of professional identity. In N. L. Chaska (Ed.), *The nursing profession: A time to speak* (pp. 134–145). New York: McGraw-Hill.

Dalton, R. J. (1996). *Citizen politics: Public opinion and political parties in advanced industrial democracies* (2nd ed.). Chatham, NJ: Chatham House Publishers.

Davies, C. (1995). *Gender and the professional predicament in nursing.* Buckingham: Open University Press.

Dawson, R. E., Prewitt, K., & Dawson, K. S. (1977). *Political socialization* (2nd ed.). Boston: Little Brown and Company.

Delevan, S. M., & Koff, S. Z. (1990). The nursing shortage and provider attitudes: A political perspective. *Journal of Public Health Policy, 11,* 62–79.

Deloughery, G. L., & Gebbie, K. M. (1975). *Political dynamics: Impact on nurses and nursing.* St. Louis: C.V. Mosby Company.

deVries, C. (1996, January/February). Poll shows SNA members more liberal than public. *The American Nurse,* p. 13.

Diers, D. (1985). Health policy and nursing curricula: A natural fit. *Nursing and Health Care, 6,* 421–433.

Dionne, E. J. (Ed.). (1998). *Community works.* Washington: Brookings Institution Press.

Driscoll, V. M. (1994). The continuing saga of nursing's failed professionalization: The New York story, 1973–1985. In D. H. Stapleton & C. A. Welch (Eds.), *Critical issues in American nursing in the twentieth century: Perspectives and case studies.* New York: Foundation of the New York State Nurses Association.

Dubar, C. (1991). *La socialisation: Construction des identités sociales et professionnelles.* Paris: Armand Colin Editeur.

Duverger, M. (1954). *Political parties: Their organization and activity in the modern state* (B. North & R. North, Trans.). New York: John Wiley & Sons.

Edwards, G. C., III, Wattenberg, M. P., & Lineberry, R. L. (2000). *Government in America: People, politics and policy* (9th ed.). New York: Longman.

Election day 1996: Your vote is critical. (1996, September). *The Report,* p. 9.

Ellis, J. R., & Hartley, C. L. (1995). *Nursing in today's world: Challenges, issues and trends* (5th ed.). Philadelphia: J. B. Lippincott.

Elzinga, A. (1990). The knowledge aspect of professionalization: The case of science-based nursing education in Sweden. In R. Torstendahl & M. Burrage (Eds.), *The formation of professions: Knowledge, state and strategy* (pp. 151–173). London: SAGE Publications.

Evans, C. L. (1995). Committees and health jurisdictions in Congress. In T. E. Mann & N. J. Ornstein (Eds.), *Intensive care: How Congress shapes health policy* (pp. 25–51). Washington: American Enterprise Institute and The Brookings Institution.

Evans, D. M. (1986). PAC contributions and roll-call voting: Conditional power. In A. J. Cigler & B. A. Loomis (Eds.), *Interest group politics* (2nd ed.). (pp. 114–132). Washington: CQ Press.

Evans, M. E. (1995). Nursing research: Influencing public policy. *Journal of the New York State Nurses Association, 26*(1), 54–56.

Evetts, J. (1999). Professional identities: State and international dynamics in engineering. In I. Hellberg, M. Saks, & C. Benoit (Eds.), *Professional identities in transition: Cross-cultural dimensions* (pp. 13–25). Göteborg: Göteborg University.

Feldman, H. R., & Lewenson, S. B. (2000). *Nurses in the political arena: The public face of nursing.* New York: Springer Publishing Company.

Feldstein, P. J. (1988). *The politics of health legislation: An economic perspective.* Ann Arbor, MI: Health Administration Press.

Fielding, A. G., & Portwood, D. (1980). Professions and the state—Towards a typology of bureaucratic professions. *The Sociological Review, 28*(1), 23–54.

Flanagan, S. (1982). Changing values in advanced industrial society. *Comparative Political Studies, 14,* 403–444.

Freidson, E. (1973). Professions and the occupational principle. In E. Freidson (Ed.), *The professions and their prospects* (pp. 19–38). Beverly Hills, CA: SAGE Publications.

Freudenheim, M., & Villarosa, L. (2001, April 8). Nursing shortage is raising worries on patients' care. *New York Times.* Retrieved April 8, 2001, from http://www.nytimes.com.

Friss, L. (1988). Simultaneous strategies for solving the nursing shortage. *Health Care Management, 13,* 71–80.

Fuller-Jonap, F. (1994). Collective bargaining in nursing: Benefits, issues, and problems. In O. L. Strickland & D. J. Fishman (Eds.), *Nursing issues in the 1990s* (pp. 33–45). Albany, NY: Delmar Publishers.

Galligan, A. C. (1985). Reaching for power from within. In R. R. Wieczorek (Ed.), *Power, politics and policy in nursing* (pp. 98–101). New York: Springer Publishing Company.

Garceau, O. (1940). Organized medicine enforces its party line. *The Public Opinion Quarterly, 4,* 408–428.

Gitelson, A. R., Conway, M. M., & Feigert, F. B. (1984). *American political parties: Stability and change.* Boston: Houghton Mifflin.

Goode, W. (1969). The theoretical limits of professionalization. In A. Etzioni (Ed.), *The semi-professions and their organization: Teachers, nurses, social workers* (pp. 266–313). New York: Free Press.

Goode, W. (1972). Community within a community: The professions. In R. M. Pavalko (Ed.), *Sociological perspectives on occupations* (pp. 17–26). Itasca, IL: F.E. Peacock Publishers.

Goodman-Draper, J. (1995). *Health care's forgotten majority: Nurses and their frayed white collars.* Westport, CT: Auburn House.

Gottlieb, L. N. (1996). Nursing in peril: A case for visibility. *Canadian Journal of Nursing Research, 28*(2), 3–5.

Greenberg, E. S., & Page, B. I. (1993). *The struggle for democracy.* New York: HarperCollins College Publishers.

Greenstein, F. I. (1972). Political socialization. In *International encyclopedia of the social sciences* (Vols. 13–14, pp. 551–555). New York: Macmillan Company and Free Press.

Greenwood, E. (1972). Attributes of a profession. In R. M. Pavalko (Ed.), *Sociological perspectives on occupations* (pp. 3–16). Itasca, IL: F.E. Peacock Publishers.

Greenwood, J. (1997). *Representing interests in the European Union.* New York: St. Martin's Press.

Grier, K. B., & Munger, M. C. (1993). Comparing interest group PAC contributions to House and Senate incumbents, 1980–1986. *The Journal of Politics, 55*(3), 615–643.

Hall, R., & Wayman, F. W. (1990). Buying time: Moneyed interests and the mobilization of bias in congressional committees. *American Political Science Review, 84*(3), 797–820.

Hall-Long, B. (1995a). Nursing education at the crossroads: Political passages. *Journal of Professional Nursing. 11*(3), 139–146.

Hall-Long, B. (1995b). Nursing's past, present, and future political experiences. *Nursing and Health Care, 16*(1), 24–28.

Hanley, B. (1983). Nurse political participation: An in-depth view and comparison with women teachers and engineers. unpublished, doctoral dissertation. University of Michigan, Ann Arbor.

Hanley, B. E. (1987). Political participation: How do nurses compare with other professional women? *Nursing Economics, 5*(4), 179–188.

Harrington, C. (1988). A policy agenda for the nursing shortage. *Nursing Outlook, 36,* 118–119, 153–154.

Hayes, E., & Fritsch, R. (1988). An untapped resource: The political potential of nurses. *Nursing Administration, 13*(1), 33–39.

Health care reform: The political arena. (1994). *Capitol Update, 12*(1), 8.

Heinz, J. P., Laumann, E. O., Salisbury, R. H., & Nelson, R. L. (1990). Inner circles or hollow cores? Elite networks in national policy systems. *Journal of Politics, 52*(2), 356–390.

Heinz, W. R. (1998). Socializzazione. In *Enciclopedia delle scienze sociali* (Vol. 8, pp. 80–89). Rome: Istituto della Enciclopedia Italiana.

Hellberg, I. (1990). The Swedish veterinary profession and the Swedish state. In R. Torstendahl & M. Burrage (Eds.), *The formation of professions: Knowledge, state and strategy* (pp. 174–185). London: SAGE Publications.

Hellberg, I., Saks, M., & Benoit, C. (1999). Introduction. In I. Hellberg, M. Saks, & C. Benoit (Eds.), *Professional identities in transition: Cross-cultural dimensions* (pp. 1–9). Göteborg: Göteborg University.

Hennessy, B. (1981). *Public opinion* (4th ed.). Monterey, CA: Brooks/Cole Publishing Company.

Hillestad, E. A., & Hawken, P. L. (1996). Nursing in the year 2000. *Journal of Professional Nursing, 12*(3), 127–128.

Hrebenar, R. J., Burbank, M. J., & Benedict, R. C. (1999). *Political parties, interest groups and campaigns.* Boulder, CO: Westview Press.

Hriceniak, J. (1994). Will the ANA survive in an era of increasing specialty organizations? In O. L. Strickland & D. J. Fishman (Eds.), *Nursing issues in the 1990s* (pp. 22–32). Albany, NY: Delmar Publishers.

Huckshorn, R. J. (1984). *Political parties in America* (2nd ed.). Monterey, CA: Brooks/Cole Publishing Company.

Iglehart, J. K. (1987). Problems facing the nursing profession. *The New England Journal of Medicine, 317,* 646–651.

Inglehart, R. (1990). *Culture shift in advanced industrial society.* Princeton: Princeton University Press.

Ingram, H., & Smith, S. (Eds.). (1993). *Public policy for democracy.* Washington: Brookings Institution.

Ippolito, D. S., Walker, T. G., & Kolson, K. L. (1976). *Public opinion and responsible democracy.* Englewood Cliffs, NJ: Prentice-Hall.

Isherwood, R. T. (1995). The curriculum revolution in nursing education: The caring perspective and its relationship to power, politics and public policy. In A. Boykin (Ed.), *Power, politics and public policy: A matter of caring* (pp. 159–177). New York: National League for Nursing Press.

Jackson, J. A. (1970). Professions and professionalization: Editorial introduction. In J. A. Jackson (Ed.), *Professions and professionalization* (pp. 3–15). London: Cambridge University Press.

Jacobs, L. R. (1993). Health reform impasse: The politics of American ambivalence toward government. *Journal of Health Politics, Policy and Law, 18*(3), 629–655.

Jacobs, L. R., & Shapiro, R. Y. (1995). Don't blame the public for failed health care reform. *Journal of Health Politics, Policy and Law, 20*(2), 411–423.

James, J. W. (Ed.). (1985). *A Lavinia Dock reader*. New York: Garland Publishing.

Jamieson, K. H., & Cappella, J. N. (1998). The role of the press in the healthcare reform debate of 1993–1994. In D. Graber, D. McQuail, & P. Norris (Eds.), *The politics of news: The news of politics* (pp. 110–131). Washington: Congressional Quarterly.

Joel, L. A. (1985). Power and the professional association. In R. R. Wieczorek (Ed.), *Power, politics and policy in nursing* (pp. 103–105). New York: Springer Publishing Company.

Jonson, K. (1998). Learning the ropes through mentoring. *The Canadian Nurse, 94*(2), 27–30.

Kalisch, B. J., & Kalisch, P. A. (1976). A discourse on the politics of nursing. *Journal of Nursing Administration, 6*(3), 29–34.

Kalisch, P. A., & Kalisch, B. J. (1995). *The advance of American nursing* (3rd ed.). Philadelphia: J.B. Lippincott.

Kaplan, M. S., & Goldberg, M. A. (1997). The media and change in health systems. In S. L. Issacs & J. R. Knickman (Eds.), *To improve health and health care* (pp. 97–108). San Francisco: Jossey-Bass.

Keepnews, D. (1998, May/June). The national sample survey of RNs: What does it tell us? *The American Nurse*, p. 10.

Kellman, K. (1998). *Outside lobbying: Public opinion and interest group strategies*. Princeton, NJ: Princeton University Press.

Kelly, L. Y., & Joel, L. A. (1995). *Dimensions of professional nursing* (7th ed.). New York: McGraw-Hill.

Kelly, L. Y., & Joel, L. A. (1996). *The nursing experience: Trends, challenges, and transitions*. New York: McGraw-Hill.

Kelly, P. M. (1999, January/February). Unity needed. *The American Nurse*, p. 4.

Kingdon, J. W. (1989). *Congressmen's voting decisions* (3rd ed.). Ann Arbor: University of Michigan Press.

Kingdon, J. W. (1995). *Agendas, alternatives, and public policy* (2nd ed.). New York: HarperCollins.

Kinsey, D. C. (1986). The new nurse influentials. *Nursing Outlook, 34*(5), 238–240.

Kosterlitz, J. (1994). Stress fractures. *National Journal, 26*(8), 412–417.

Krantzler, N. J. (1986). Media images of physicians and nurses in the United States. *Social Science and Medicine, 22*(9), 933–952.

Krause, E. A. (1998). The politics of professional expertise. In V. Olgiati, L. Orzack, & M. Saks (Eds.), *Professions, identity, and order in com-*

parative perspective (pp. 365–378). Onati: The International Institute for the Sociology of Law.

Kuhn, R. (1986). Strength in numbers: Will we use it? *Heart and Lung, 15*(1), 24A–27A.

LaChat, M. R. (1988). Religion's support for the domination of women—Breaking the cycle. *Nurse Practitioner, 13*(1), 31–34.

Ladd, E. C. (1999). *The Ladd report.* New York: Free Press.

Larson, M. S. (1977). *The rise of professionalism: A sociological analysis.* Berkeley, CA: University of California Press.

Larson, M. S. (1990). In the matter of experts and professionals, or how impossible it is to leave nothing unsaid. In R. Torstendahl & M. Burrage (Eds.), *The formation of professions: Knowledge, state and strategy* (pp. 24–50). London: SAGE Publications.

Leavitt, J. K. (1994). Policy and politics—A necessity for inclusion in nursing curricula: Our nursing practice depends on it. *Dean's Notes, 16*(2), 1–3.

Leavitt, J. K., & Mason, D. J. (1994). Finding your political voice. *American Journal of Nursing, 94*(10), 56–58.

Leggatt, T. (1970). Teaching as a profession. In J. A. Jackson (Ed.), *Professions and professionalization* (pp. 155–177). London: Cambridge University Press.

Lerner, H. M. (1985). Educating nurses for power. In R. R. Wieczorek (Ed.), *Power, politics and policy in nursing* (pp. 90–94). New York: Springer Publishing Company.

Levi, M. (1980). Functional redundancy and the process of professionalization: The case of registered nurses in the United States. *Journal of Health Politics, Policy and Law, 5*(2), 333–353.

Levi, M. (1995). Functional redundancy and the process of professionalization: The case of registered nurses in the United States. In W. G. Rothstein (Ed.), *Readings in American health care: Current issues in sociohistorical perspective* (pp. 199–211). Madison: University of Wisconsin Press.

Levinson, R. M., McCranie, E. W., Scambler, G., & Scambler, A. (1995). Physician authority and the autonomy of nurses and patients: Attitudes of British and U.S. medical students. *Research in the Sociology of Health Care, 12,* 355–368.

Lewenson, S. B. (1993). *Taking charge: Nursing, suffrage, and feminism in America, 1873–1920.* New York: Garland Publishing.

Lewis, M. D. (1985). The academic power of nursing deans. In R. R. Wieczorek (Ed.), *Power, politics and policy* (pp. 174–187). New York: Springer Publishing Company.

Lindblom, C. E. (1968). *The policy-making process.* Englewood Cliffs, NJ: Prentice-Hall.

Lowery-Palmer, A. (1982). The cultural basis of political behavior in two groups: Nurses and political activists . In J. Muff (Ed.), *Socialization, sexism, and stereotyping: Women's issues in nursing* (pp. 189–202). St. Louis: C.V. Mosby Company.

Lucco, J. (1992). Representing the public interest: Consumer groups and the presidency. In M. P. Petracca (Ed.), *The politics of interests: Interest groups transformed* (pp. 242–262). Boulder, CO: Westview Press.

Lynaugh, J. E., & Brush, B. L. (1996). *American nursing: From hospitals to health systems.* Cambridge, MA: Blackwell Publishers.

Lynn, M. R., McCain, N. L., & Boss, B. J. (1989). Socialization of RN to BSN. *Image: Journal of Nursing Scholarship, 21*(4), 232–237.

Macdonald, K. M. (1995). *The sociology of the professions.* London: SAGE Publications.

Malone, B. L. (1998, May/June). Professionalism: An exercise in stretching. *The American Nurse,* p. 5.

Manley, J. E. (1995). Sex-segregated work in the system of professions: The development and stratification of nursing. *The Sociological Quarterly, 36*(2), 297–314.

Mann, T. E., & Ornstein, N. J. (1995). Introduction. In T. E. Mann & N. J. Ornstein (Eds.), *Intensive care: How Congress shapes health policy* (pp. 1–22). Washington: American Enterprise Institute and Brookings Institution.

Maraldo, P. (1985). The illusion of power. In R. R. Wieczorek (Ed.), *Power, politics and policy in nursing* (pp. 64–73). New York: Springer Publishing Company.

Martin, E. J., White, J. E., & Hansen, M. (1989). Preparing students to shape health policy. *Nursing Outlook, 37,* 89–94.

Mason, D. J. (1990). Nursing and politics: A profession comes of age. *Orthopaedic Nursing, 9*(5), 11–17.

Mason, D. J., & Leavitt, J. K. (1995). Political activism: The individual versus the collective. *Journal of the New York State Nurses Association, 26*(1), 46–47.

McCarthy, C. (1988, July 24). The wrong prescription for hospital care. *The Washington Post.*

McClelland, C. E. (1991). *The German experience of professionalization.* Cambridge: Cambridge University Press.

McCullough, C. (1995). Collective bargaining: Empowerment and change. *Journal of the New York State Nurses Association, 26*(1), 44–45.

McIntosh, D. (1989). Grassroots lobbying. *American Journal of Nursing, 89*(11), 1515–1516.

The medical profession: It hurts. (1999, February 6). *The Economist,* pp. 52–53.

Membership matters. (1995, January/February). *The American Nurse,* p. 14.

Merton, R. K. (1957). Some preliminaries to a sociology of medical education. In R. K. Merton, G. Reader, & P. L. Kendall (Eds.), *The student physician* (pp. 3–79). Cambridge, MA: Harvard University Press.

Milbrath, L., & Goel, M. L. (1977). *Political participation.* New York: Rand McNally.

Milio, N. (1989). Developing nursing leadership in health policy. *Journal of Professional Nursing, 5*(6), 315–321.

Milio, N. B. (1985). Nursing within the ecology of public policy: A case in point. In R. White (Ed.), *Political issues in nursing: Past, present and future* (pp. 87–104). Chichester: John Wiley & Sons.

Moe, T. M. (1980). *The organization of interests.* Chicago: University of Chicago Press.

Montgomery, B. (1994). Caregiver education: Feminist or male model? *Health Care for Women International, 15*(6), 481–488.

Mueller, K. J. (1993). *Health care policy in the United States.* Lincoln: University of Nebraska Press.

National Advisory Council on Nurse Education and Practice. (2000). *Report to the Secretary of Health and Human Services and Congress: A national agenda for nursing workforce—Racial/ethnic diversity.* Washington: U.S. Department of Health and Human Services.

National Commission on Nursing. (1988). *Final report.* Washington: Department of Health and Human Services.

National labor entity: United American Nurses. Retrieved July 19, 2000, from http://www.nursingworld.org.

National League for Nursing. (1995). *Nurse educators 1995: Findings from the RN and LPN faculty census.* New York: National League for Nursing.

The nation's nurses: A credible profession doing an incredible job. (1988). Milwaukee, WI: National Commission on Nursing Implementation Project.

New nursing data. (1997, April 25). *Capitol Update, 15*(6), 6.

Nurses missing from media coverage. (1998, January/February). *The American Nurse,* p. 21.

Nursing supporters elected to U.S. Congress. (2000, November/December). *The American Nurse*, p. 3.

Olesen, V., & Whittaker, E. W. (1970). Critical notes on sociological studies of professional socialization. In J. A. Jackson (Ed.), *Professions and professionalization* (pp. 181–221). London: Cambridge University Press.

Oliver, P. E., & Maney, G. M. (2000). Political processes and local newspaper coverage of protest events: From selection bias to triadic interactions. *American Journal of Sociology, 106*(2), 463–505.

Olson, M. (1965). *The logic of collective action*. Cambridge, MA: Harvard University Press.

Orsolits, M., Frainer, M., Haughey, B., Stanton, M., Kimsley, M., Eddins, E., et al. (1983). Nurses' knowledge about and attitudes toward professional nursing organizations. *Journal of the New York State Nurses Association, 14*(4), 32–40.

Paletz, D. L. (1998). The media and public policy. In D. Graber, D. McQuail, & P. Norris (Eds.), *The politics of news: The news of politics* (pp. 218–237). Washington: Congressional Quarterly.

Palmer, I. S. (1983). From whence we came. In N. L. Chaska (Ed.), *The nursing profession: A time to speak* (pp. 3–28). New York: McGraw-Hill.

Patel, K., & Rushefsky, M. E. (1995). *Health care politics and policy in America*. Armonk, NY: M.E. Sharpe.

Pavalko, R. M. (1971). *Sociology of occupations and professions*. Itasca, IL: F.E. Peacock Publishers.

Pease, J. (1972). Faculty influence and professional participation of doctoral students. In R. M. Pavalko (Ed.), *Sociological perspectives on occupations* (pp. 177–185). Itasca, IL: F.E. Peacock Publishers.

Perrucci, R. (1973). Engineering: Professional servant in power. In E. Freidson (Ed.), *The professions and their prospects* (pp. 119–133). Beverly Hills, CA: SAGE Publications.

Peterson, M. A. (1992). The presidency and organized interests: White House patterns of interest group liaison. *American Political Science Review, 86*(3), 612–625.

Peterson, M. A. (1993). Political influence in the 1990s: From iron triangles to policy networks. *Journal of Health Politics, Policy and Law, 18*(2), 395–438.

Petracca, M. P. (1992). The rediscovery of interest group politics. In M. P. Petracca (Ed.), *The politics of interests: Interest groups transformed* (pp. 3–31). Boulder, CO: Westview Press.

Pew Health Professions Commission. (1993). *Health professions education for the future: Schools in service to the nation.* San Francisco, CA: Pew Health Professions Commission.

Pew Health Professions Commission. (1995). *Critical challenges: Revitalizing the health professions for the twenty-first century.* San Francisco, CA: UCSF Center for the Health Professions.

Political update. (1998, October 31). *Capitol Update, 16*(18), 5–7.

Purposes outlined for new councils. (1994, February). *The American Nurse,* pp. 10–11.

Putnam, R. D. (2000). *Bowling alone.* New York: Simon & Schuster.

Rains, J. W. (1988). Nursing and politics: Adapting skills to spark social change. *Nursing and Health Care, 9*(6), 299–301.

Ramprogus, V. (1995). *The deconstruction of nursing.* Aldershot: Avebury.

Raudonis, B. M., & Griffith, H. (1991). Model for integrating health services research and health care policy formation. *Nursing and Health Care, 12*(1), 32–36.

Roberts, J. I., & Group, T. M. (1995). *Feminism and nursing: An historical perspective on power, status and political activism in the nursing profession.* Westport, CT: Praeger Publishers.

Romer, T., & Snyder, J. M., Jr. (1994). An empirical investigation of the dynamics of PAC contributions. *American Journal of Political Science, 38*(3), 745–769.

Rosella, J. D., Regan-Kubinski, M. J., & Albrecht, S. A. (1994). The need for multicultural diversity among health professionals. *Nursing and Health Care, 15*(5), 242–246.

Rothberg, J. S. (1985). The growth of political action in nursing: The formation of N-CAP began a new chapter in nursing's political history. *Nursing Outlook, 33*(3), 133–135.

Ruby, J. (1998). Baccalaureate nurse educators' workload and productivity: Ascription of values and the challenges of evaluation. *The Journal of the New York State Nurses Association, 29*(2), 18–22.

Rueschemeyer, D. (1993). Professional autonomy and the social control expertise. In R. Dingwall & P. Lewis (Eds.), *The sociology of the professions: Lawyer, doctors and others* (pp. 38–58). New York: St. Martin's Press.

Sabatier, P. A. (1992). Interest group membership and organization: Multiple theories. In M. P. Petracca (Ed.), *The politics of interests: Interest groups transformed* (pp. 99–129). Boulder, CO: Westview Press.

Saks, M. (1999). Towards integrated health care: Shifting professional interests and identities in Britain. In I. Hellberg, M. Saks, & C. Benoit (Eds.), *Professional identities in transition: Cross-cultural dimensions* (pp. 295–309). Göteborg: Göteborg University.

Salisbury, R. H., Heinz, J. P., Laumann, E. O., & Nelson, R. L. (1987). Who works with whom? Interest group alliances and opposition. *American Political Science Review, 81*(4), 1217–1234.

Schick, A. (1995). How a bill did not become a law. In T. E. Mann & N. J. Ornstein (Eds.), *Intensive care: How Congress shapes health policy* (pp. 227–272). Washington: American Enterprise Institute and Brookings Institution.

Schlozman, K. L., & Tierney, J. T. (1986). *Organized interests and American democracy.* New York: HarperCollins.

Schutzenhofer, K. K., & Musser, D. B. (1994). Nurse characteristics and professional autonomy. *Image, 26*(3), 201–205.

Seelye, K. Q. (1994, August 16). Lobbyists are the loudest in the health care debate. *New York Times,* pp. A1, A12.

Serafini, M. W. (1995). Who's in charge here? *National Journal, 27*(26), 1710–1713.

Sharp, N., Biggs, S., & Wakefield, M. (1991). Public policy: New opportunities for nurses. *Nursing and Health Care, 12*(1), 16–22.

Shaver, J. L. F. (1994, February). What the new council structure means for you. *The American Nurse,* pp. 10–11.

Sherwin, L. N. (1998). When the mission is teaching: Does nursing faculty practice fit? *Journal of Professional Nursing, 14*(3), 137–143.

Shields, T. G., & Goidel, R. K. (2000). Who contributes? Checkbook participation, class biases and the impact of legal reforms, 1952–1994. *American Politics Quarterly, 28*(2), 216–233.

Simpson, I. H. (1972). Patterns of socialization into professions: The case of student nurses. In R. M. Pavalko (Ed.), *Sociological perspectives on occupations* (pp. 169–177). Itasca, IL: F.E. Peacock Publishers.

Skocpol, T., Ganz, M., & Munson, Z. (2000). A nation of organizers: The institutional origins of civic voluntarism in the United States. *American Political Science Review, 94*(3), 527–546.

Smith, D. A. (1998). *Tax crusaders and the politics of direct democracy.* New York: Routledge.

Smith, R. A. (1995). Interest group influence in the U.S. Congress. *Legislative Studies Quarterly, 20*(1), 89–139.

Smith, S. R. (1995). The role of institutions and ideas in health care policy. *Journal of Health Politics, Policy and Law, 20*(2), 385–389.

Smolowitz, J., & Murray, M. F. (1997). Nursing research activities in New York State are alive and well: A survey of selected acute care facilities and schools of nursing. *Journal of the New York State Nurses Association, 28*(3), 20–23.

SNA members see country doing well, quality of health care declining. (1999, January/February). *The American Nurse*, p.17.

Solomons, H. C., Jordison, N. S., & Powell, S. R. (1980). How faculty members spend their time. *Nursing Outlook, 28*(3), 160–165.

Sower, M. M. (1996). Annual report of the State Board for Nursing. *Report, 27*(10), 5–7.

Speak up. (1994, April). *The American Nurse*, p. 19.

Spradley, B. W., & Allender, J. A. (1996). *Community health nursing: Concepts and practice* (4th ed.). Philadelphia: Lippincott.

Starr, P. (1994). *The logic of health care reform: Why and how the President's plan will work* (Rev. ed.). New York: Whittle Books in association with Penguin Books.

Stern, P. M. (1988). *The best Congress money can buy.* New York: Pantheon.

Stimpson, M., & Hanley, B. (1991). Nurse policy analyst: Advanced practice role. *Nursing and Health Care, 12*(1), 10–15.

Strauss, G. (1963). Professionalism and occupational associations. *Industrial Relations, 2*(3), 21.

Thomas, P. A., & Shelton, C. R. (1994). Teaching students to become active in public policy. *Public Health Nursing, 11*(2), 75–79.

The top 10 PACS. (1996, November 3). *Parade Magazine*, p. 13.

Torstendahl, R. (1990). Introduction: Promotion and strategies of knowledge-based groups. In R. Torstendahl & M. Burrage (Eds.), *The formation of professions: Knowledge, state and strategy* (pp. 1–10). London: SAGE Publications.

Tousijn, W. (1997). Professioni. In *Enciclopedia delle scienze sociali* (Vol. 7, pp. 48–57). Rome: Istituto dell'Enciclopedia Italiana.

Tousijn. W. (2000). *Il sistema delle occupazioni sanitarie.* Bologna: Il Mulino.

25 years later. (1990). *The Nurse Practitioner, 15*(9), 9–28.

United States. In Roger East (Vol. Ed.), *Keesing's record of world events:* Vol. 42 (11) *News digest* (1996, November, pp. 41357–41360). Cambridge, England: Keesing's Worldwide.

United States. In D. S. Lewis (Vol. Ed.), *Keesing's record of world events:* Vol. 46 (11) *News digest* (2000, November, pp. 43841–43847). Cambridge, England: Keesing's Worldwide.

Vollmer, H. M., & Mills, D. L. (Eds.). (1966). *Professionalization.* Englewood Cliffs, NJ: Prentice Hall.

Walby, S., & Greenwell, J. (1994). *Medicine and nursing: Professions in a changing health service.* London: SAGE Publications.

Walker, J. L. (1983). The origins and maintenance of interest groups in America. *American Political Science Review, 77*(2), 390–406.

Waters, M. (1989). Patriarchy and viriarchy: An exploration and reconstruction of concepts of masculine domination. *Sociology, 23*(2), 193–211.

Weissert, C. S., & Weissert, W. G. (1996). *Governing health: The politics of health policy.* Baltimore: Johns Hopkins University Press.

Welch, C. A. (1985). Nursing, policy, and the association. In R. R. Wieczorek (Ed.), *Power, politics and policy in nursing* (pp. 106–113). New York: Springer Publishing Company.

White House Domestic Policy Council. (n.d.). *Health security: The President's report to the American people.* New York: Touchstone.

Williamson, J. A. (1983). Crisis in academic nursing. In N. L. Chaska (Ed.), *The nursing profession: A time to speak* (pp. 63–69). New York: McGraw-Hill.

Wilsford, D. (1991). *Doctors and the state: The politics of health care in France and the United States.* Durham, NC: Duke University Press.

Witz, A. (1992). *Professions and patriarchy.* London: Routledge.

Wolinsky, H., & Brune, T. (1994). *The serpent on the staff: The unhealthy politics of the American Medical Association.* New York: G. P. Putnam's Sons.

Zerwekh, J., & Claborn, J. C. (1994). *Nursing today: Transition and trends.* Philadelphia: W.B. Saunders.

Zuckerman, E. (Ed.). (1998). *The almanac of federal PACs: 1998–99.* Arlington, VA: Amward Publications.

Index